International Perspectives on Aging

Volume 39

The study of aging is continuing to increase rapidly across multiple disciplines. This wide-ranging series on International Perspectives on Aging provides readers with much-needed comprehensive texts and critical perspectives on the latest research, policy, and practical developments. Both aging and globalization have become a reality of our times, yet a systematic effort of a global magnitude to address aging is yet to be seen. The series bridges the gaps in the literature and provides cutting-edge debate on new and traditional areas of comparative aging, all from an international perspective. More specifically, this book series on International Perspectives on Aging puts the spotlight on international and comparative studies of aging.

Satya Brink

The Longevity Dividend

Later Life, Lifelong Learning and Productive Societies

Springer

Satya Brink
International advisor – Policy research
Chelsea, QC, Canada

ISSN 2197-5841 ISSN 2197-585X (electronic)
International Perspectives on Aging
ISBN 978-3-031-35334-5 ISBN 978-3-031-35335-2 (eBook)
https://doi.org/10.1007/978-3-031-35335-2

This Springer imprint is published by the registered company Springer Nature Switzerland AG
The registered company address is: Gewerbestrasse 11, 6330 Cham, Switzerland

To Lars
My partner in love, learning and life

Foreword

Lifelong learning is again moving up the political agenda. This is, in my experience, something that happens roughly every decade: politicians or journalists or researchers discover that it is a good idea for people to have the opportunity to learn at any age, rather than just in their first two or three decades. The arguments are usually sound; the problem is to make them stick, such that they gain traction in a world where education is still so strongly seen as synonymous with youth.

Demographic change is one of the most powerful drivers behind the most recent awareness of the merits of lifelong learning. Across the globe populations are ageing. This trend presents challenges and opportunities: challenges most obviously in sustaining the health and wellbeing of older people, but also in myriad other forms which involve the whole population; and opportunities which are there to be grasped in enabling people of all ages to make the most of the additional years that most of them will live.

However, as Satya Brink points out, the trend may be almost universal but it is far from uniform. Most OECD countries are well down the ageing route, with older people forming a growing proportion of their populations. In other parts of the world, people are also living longer, but the potential longevity dividend takes different forms as the process starts from further back and/or the numbers of young people continue to increase. Similarly, the general case for lifelong learning holds across all societies, but the specific form it takes will vary from country to country. As Brink eloquently says, learning is 'a mutual responsibility and a collective obligation'. It is for each society to work out the most appropriate way to give practical reality to the rhetoric of lifelong learning. That said, international comparisons of the kind enabled by this book are an invaluable tool for learning from each other and therefore arriving at solutions which yield the most positive results.

If we are to achieve systemic change in the direction of lifelong learning, Brink argues, we need to think about the overall infrastructure across the full life course. I agree, including on the need for better and more dynamic modelling of the life course, rather than simplistic linear models which are too tightly linked to chronological age. Drawing on her experience in national and international government agencies, she directs attention to the range of roles which government needs to occupy. These include leadership, coordination and quality assurance, but I would especially emphasize the need for effective and continuing evidence generation. This involves not just systematic monitoring and data gathering, but assembling different kinds of evidence to build a complete picture which evolves over time. Longitudinal evidence is particularly important here. (One of the recommendations we made 12 years ago in the final report of the UK's Inquiry into the Future of Lifelong Learning was for a biennial or triennial Review of the Nation's Learning, which would supply a regular and cumulative stocktake of progress – or lack of it.)

Brink's book is a broad-ranging articulation of the need to take advantage of current trends. As she says, we are witnessing a unique transition, and if we do not move to take advantage, it will be more than just a missed opportunity for older people. A crucial benefit of genuine lifelong learning is the way it fosters intergenerational communication and understanding – arguably something needed more than ever in these days of siloed social media. Economic, health and social effects are all intertwined, which is exactly why we need the kind of extensive canvas this book provides.

Tom Schuller
Former Head of OECD's Centre for Educational Research and Innovation; author of *The Paula Principle: Why Women's Competences Are Undervalued* (Scribe 2017) and principal editor of UNESCO's 3rd Global Report on Adult Learning and Education (2016).

Abstract

Can society benefit from an ageing population? This book explains how current and future generations can benefit from the longevity dividend in the coming decades, using multidisciplinary and international evidence.

How? It depends on the strategic choices of countries. And if they act before the opportunity closes. Growing life expectancy will increase the active years of later life by 25 years or more, resulting in more than a quarter of the population aged over 65 years in many countries. The social, economic and cultural impacts of this phenomenon are massive as the population shifts from a youthful population to one with a large older population. This population structure includes a greater number of adults with knowledge and skills than before that can contribute to society compared to fewer adults living shorter lives. Their contributions can be economically and socially productive by increasing growth, reducing costs as well as advancing social progress. The longevity dividend is realized because the total contributions of societal and economic value increase because there are more citizens contributing during longer lives. The longevity dividend is the windfall gain in economic growth and social progress gained during this once only population shift. Society retains this gain and then continues growth from the peak benefitting future generations. The two ways to increase the dividend are to increase the total contributions that benefit society and to improve the quality of these contributions over the lifetime of citizens through lifelong learning. Increased contributions during the prolonged lives of the entire population result in a productive society. Informed countries will make deliberate choices to gain a greater longevity dividend during this one-time opportunity to benefit from greater life expectancy.

Acknowledgements

It is with deep gratitude that I acknowledge my colleagues and friends in governments, academia, institutions, international organizations and the non-profit sector who encouraged and promoted the development of ideas that I present in this book.

Contents

List of Figures

List of Tables

About the Author

Satya Brink personally knows about later life. She is an internationally known researcher, author and policy advisor in the field of learning, both in its component parts and as a lifelong endeavour. She was a Director of National Policy Research on Learning for the Canadian government creating evidence with her team for public policy. She has worked for international organizations such as the Organization for Economic Cooperation and Development (OECD), World Bank, the United Nations Educational, Scientific and Cultural Organization (UNESCO) and the UNESCO Institute for Lifelong Learning (UIL). As an international consultant, she has conducted work for a range of governments in developed and developing countries, such as Finland, Ireland, Senegal and Egypt. She was an adjunct Professor of Gerontology at Simon Fraser University in Canada and is currently associated with the Lifelong Learning Institute ENCELL at Jönköping University in Sweden.

About the Author

[illegible]

Chapter 1
Life Expectancy, Learning in Later Life and the Longevity Dividend

1.1 The Global Longevity Phenomenon

To your long life! Wishes for a long life have been a widely used blessing in many cultures around the world. Long life was relatively rare for centuries. But in this century, longevity is growing widely around the globe for the first time in human history. In every age cohort more people have lived longer than before, at least since 1950 (Fig. 1.1). Average world life expectancy at birth grew by 24 years from 47.7 years in 1960 to 71.7 in 2022 (Population Division, 2022a). While the United Nations estimates that in 2020 there were 152 million people over the age of 80 years in the world, it projects this age cohort to triple to 459 million by 2050. Better health, more education and higher standards of living contribute to the growth in longevity. The longevity phenomenon is both an exceptional achievement and a unique experience for humanity.

In developed countries, the aging baby boomers are now part of the growing numbers of older people. Greater longevity is expected to continue to extend life in the twenty-first century. The share of the global population 65 and over is projected to rise from 10% in 2022 to 16% in 2050 (Population Division, 2022b). Those born in 2018 in developed countries may live as long as 90 years, or even 100 years.

The growing life expectancy that causes population aging around the world results in extra years of life, which means the later years become a much longer and more diverse phase of life. The later years offer a longer time for self-actualization and productive contributions to society. Existing notions of old age no longer adequately describe this age group or the process of aging in the later years. There are moral, economic and social reasons to ensure that both older people and the society to which they belong become beneficiaries of this demographic change.

S. Brink, *The Longevity Dividend*, International Perspectives on Aging 39,
https://doi.org/10.1007/978-3-031-35335-2_1

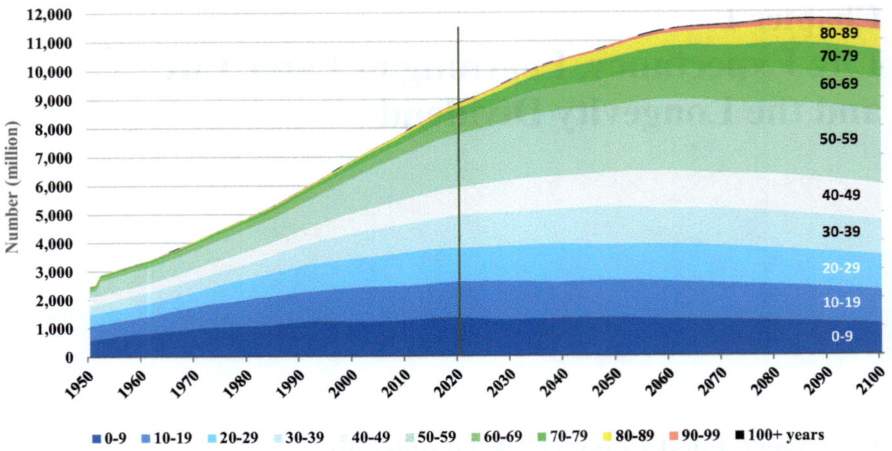

Fig. 1.1 World population projections of 10-year age cohorts showing growth in older population between 1950 and 2100. (Data from Population Division (2022c, Population by 5-year age groups and sex, World), © 2022 United Nations, with permission from the United Nations)

1.2 Learning for Worthwhile Extra Years of Life

Earlier, the later years of life were considered a period of decline and deficits leading to death, so aging was not associated with learning. Since people rarely lived as long as a hundred years, there was no thought about learning to gain the most from these decades in the later years for both successful personal aging and the prosperity of society. The learning system was built to educate the younger generations to prepare them for work. It was not designed to engage older people in learning for successful aging in later life.

Traditionally greater age was associated with wisdom. There is some empirical evidence that social wisdom improves with age because older people tend to seek compromise in competing options and use more complex reasoning and multiple perspectives (Grossman et al., 2010). However, there is also evidence to show that they do not engage in learning in their later years and are not up to date with new technologies. Why don't people in their later years continue to learn as they did when they were younger?

Rights to learning can no longer exclude such a large and experienced population segment. The purpose of learning is to grow and thrive; not just for careers nor just for recreation in old age. Human beings are learning machines and they stop learning only if they are prevented from doing so. Lifelong learning does not end at the termination of working years – it rather continues to enrich lives until the end. But lifelong learning faces challenges in meeting the needs of people throughout a much longer lifespan, challenges in terms of access, design, content, delivery and assessment.

Learning helps to improve the aging experience and increase participation in society. In addition, learning by individuals helps them to contribute to goals larger than themselves, which improves the lives of others and the state of the world. Learning results in foresight by cultivating the ability to hypothesize a relationship between two or more events separated by time (Davis, 1986). Humans, unlike other species, can thus aspire and plan for their own wellbeing as well as that of the future of society.

The general value of lifelong learning is unchanged throughout life though the objective of learning and its planned use, choice of content and means may vary depending on age and circumstances. There are intrinsic as well as instrumental reasons why humans instinctively engage in learning. Intrinsic learning is valued for its own sake, wisdom as an end in itself and for the pleasure of learning. Instrumental learning is valued for the end results gained from its use. These values need not be mutually exclusive and learning may involve both. Though most learning is intentional, incidental or unplanned learning can occur from lived experience or as a byproduct of formal learning. People do not always analyze all potential purposes of knowledge before learning, but they instinctively know when to apply the specific things that they have learned where the situation demands this particular knowledge or skill. Table 1.1 outlines common purposes for intrinsic and instrumental learning, which range from work to pleasure.

1.3 Lifelong Learning Builds Human Capital for the Benefit of Individuals and Nations

Learning is the process by which human capital is amassed. Human capital is the accumulated personal stock of knowledge, skills and attributes (including leadership and creativity) that a person can use in everyday life as well as to achieve future goals. Human capital is updated and accumulated throughout life. By transmitting their human capital, people share their human capital with others who build on the endowment. This process passes on valuable human capital from generation to generation, resulting in societal wealth gained from applied knowledge, know-how, time savings, innovation, security and psychological wellbeing.

Human capital is multidimensional and may be the aggregate of knowledge, skills and attributes related to specific domains of daily life. Therefore, human capital has to be built, used and transmitted even in later life. The components of human capital are inter-related.

1.3.1 Knowledge Capital

Knowledge capital, also referred to as intellectual capital, is the development of mental frameworks, information and tacit knowledge which can include facts, relationships, procedures and techniques as well as new ideas. Such factual, conceptual, procedural and metacognitive knowledge is essential for problem solving, logical

Table 1.1 The value of lifelong learning at all ages of life

Value of lifelong learning at all ages of life		
Value	Type of purpose	Description
Intrinsic, valued for its own sake	Life awareness	To understand the world in which life is lived – its geography, history, culture, current events and life context
	Learning for 'brain cleaning' and pleasure	To unlearn for brain cleaning, relearn or upgrade To learn new things for the pleasure of learning
Instrumental, valued for the potential end results	Knowledge for productive personal decisions	To reach the fullest potential of one's life To cope with a rapidly changing world and environment by up-to-date knowledge To create new knowledge to share and use for future benefit
	Knowledge and skills for work	To gain expertise and professional knowledge for work and employment To use current technologies for quality of life and communication To make a satisfying difference through one's life and to change things for the better
	Life and people skills	To analytically evaluate and critically think to solve new and unexpected problems in personal life or society To learn new knowledge, skills and practices to adapt to the natural and social environment To work with others for mutual benefit

Author's elaboration (2023)

thinking and reasoned argument. It provides the basis for wise decisions and choices that benefit the individual, family, community and society. It is the ability to generate ideas, create and innovate from a solid knowledge base.

1.3.2 Health Capital

Health capital relates to the sense of energy, strength, vitality and stamina of individuals that contribute to well-being, productivity and longevity (Arrow et al., 2014). Health capital is strongly interrelated with other types of capital.

1.3.3 Social Capital

Social capital is gained from social networks and the skill in developing and using them. These social assets consist of the relationships, links, shared values and collective information in society that enable individuals and groups to trust each other and work together for common purposes and societal harmony (Organisation for Economic Co-operation and Development [OECD] & Centre for Educational Research and Innovation [CERI], 2007). Social networks and interactions can depend on the type of social capital relationships (Woolcock, 2001). Bonding social capital links like-minded people in similar situations. Bridging social capital is the connections between heterogeneous groups – connections may be fragile but can foster social inclusion. Linking social capital is the relationship between unlike people in dissimilar situations, often entirely outside the community. Social capital is particularly aided by social media and the internet, where individuals can leverage a wider range of resources than are available in their own community within close geographical proximity.

1.3.4 Civic Capital

Civic capital comprises the understanding of one's place in society and the world as a global citizen. It is a sense of belonging, civic duty and social participation, which encourages volunteering for improving the conditions of others in the community and also in the world. It is the public-spirited ability to work together with others or with organizations in an ad hoc, voluntary or formal way to solve problems that have a wide impact.

1.3.5 Financial Capital

Financial capital is the money, credit, property and assets that constitute the economic resources of the individual. It is also the ability to manage prudent consumption, careful saving and wise investments. Financial capital increases the opportunities to gain other types of capital.

1.3.6 Cultural Capital

Cultural capital is the use of knowledge, behaviours and skills that can demonstrate cultural competence and social status when working with others or in the community. Cultural capital promotes social mobility and social relations in society (Bourdieu, 1973). Cultural capital may be a source of knowledge capital gained from literature and the arts.

1.3.7 Life Capital

Though not always recognized, life capital is the store of life skills that enable individuals to gain the most from life experiences and to cope with positive and negative life events. It gives individuals the confidence to transform life force into tangible results and legacy actions.

Learning results in a dynamic stock of human capital, where individuals discard less useful knowledge and skills through a process of brain cleaning and gain new ones that are more pertinent to current and future needs. Such learning can occur through formal processes such as education and training or self-learning through life experiences and through interaction with others. The knowledge, skills and attributes can also be improved through practice, emulating models and experts and by trial and error. These learning skills are honed throughout life.

The returns to learning, education and training may not be immediate but these processes provide durable returns in the long term. Learning results in both private returns and social returns. Adam Smith in the eighteenth century already recognized the national value of the acquired knowledge and talents of all inhabitants in society. Prosperity and quality of life are created by the ingenuity, innovation and effort of a country's population.

Private returns go primarily to an individual and can be measured both as monetary returns and in terms of quality of life. Such private monetary returns arise from better employability, better jobs and higher earnings. Higher status and larger networks are related to more opportunities in life. Quality of life returns include improved health and a longer life span. Research from the United States found that an additional four years of education lowers five-year mortality by 1.8 percentage points (Cutler & Lleras-Muney, 2006). It also reduces the risk of heart disease by 2.2 percentage points and the risk of diabetes by 1.3 percentage points. Adults with higher levels of foundation skills (literacy and numeracy) had a higher likelihood of better health. They participate more in community groups and organizations and they feel they can make a difference in social and political life (OECD, 2016).

The human capital of individuals collectively contributes to the national human capital, which is essential for economic growth, prosperity and standard of living. While financial capital and natural capital also contribute, human capital is responsible for productive labour, technological advancement, community engagement, civic participation, consumption and national growth. The rate of national development is dependent on the growth in national human capital.

Society also benefits from increased social returns to human capital resulting from a knowledgeable productive labour force, better population health outcomes, lower levels of crime, cleaner environment and generally better governance. Raising national human capital through learning initiates a virtuous cycle, since healthy well-informed people with few stressors in their lives tend to be more productive and contributing members of society (Keeley, 2007). A nation's social progress is thus also dependent on well utilized collective human capital.

1.4 Investing in Learning Throughout Life

Lifelong learning, including in the later years, enables older people to do what they value, retain the ability to make decisions, preserve their identity in society and maintain independence in their lives. There is no justification to stop learning at the end of working life. Lifelong learning allows individuals to achieve their maximum potential throughout life. Learning helps them to build their human capital for their own life achievement goals, to make their societal contributions better and to consider their legacy to future generations.

Nurturing human capital in all individuals as they live longer is essential for national economic growth and societal wellbeing. Investing in learning is both an individual and societal long-term strategy. Continuous learning through life is a vital way to ensure that the members of the population are ready and able to use their knowledge and skills to tackle the personal and national challenges of their lifetimes.

Lack of learning leads to negative outcomes resulting from a vicious cycle. Since learning affects behaviours as well as results, uninformed people can intentionally or unintentionally engage in activities that result in poor health, lower incomes and social exclusion. In the long run, greater human capital reduces the cost of these societal disadvantages, especially if the returns to learning are well distributed among all parts of the population. Investing in human capital is the single most effective strategy for promoting national growth and distributing its benefits, both economic and social, more fairly among all societal groups.

1.5 Later Years – Blessing or Burden?

There is a prevailing societal misconception that people in their later years are a burden to their families and to society because of age related decline. The minority that are frail or demented may be dependent, passive recipients of care and incapable of making decisions. Unfortunately, they form the stereotype for a vibrant majority of people who actively contribute while living healthy lives to an advanced age. These negative views interfere in the potential for persons in their later years to participate in and contribute to society. The idea that the later years are always years of decline is based on partial and faulty evaluation of current reality. There is an inverse relationship between autonomy and the need for care and social protection. If society invests in autonomy for as many people and for as long as possible, the social and public costs will decline and their contributions will rise. Opportunities for participation are a guarantee against costly social exclusion of people in their later years. There should be no doubt that growing old is a blessing now given to many more than before.

The life course perspective views healthy aging as a lifelong process. Social contributions wax and wane and change in content and extent according to one's age, roles and situation through one's lifetime. These contributions do not necessarily peak in early adulthood or progressively decline in older years. This phenomenon is described as contributive justice, where it is the responsibility of each society member, regardless of stage in life, to contribute to the function and wellbeing of society. It is considered just because it matches expectations of contributions with the capabilities in an individual's stage of life (Sandel, 2020). People in the later years of life have diversified human capital, depending on when and what they learned over their lifetime, which affects their contributions. With the varied human capital and experience built over a long lifetime, older people continue to contribute and even work as active agents of change for society and future generations. The value of the later years of life can be a positive force for the good of society through the longevity dividend, making long lives a blessing rather than a burden.

1.6 The Longevity Dividend Benefits Living and Future Generations

Growing life expectancy offers an unanticipated opportunity for greater social prosperity. The transition from a population structure with a high proportion of children to one with a high proportion of older people results from people living longer. Society gains from a longer life expectancy because it increases the pool of potentially productive adults capable of contributions that benefit society. Older people have a longer lifetime of knowledge and experience which, when added rather than ignored, can increase the quantity and quality of the total contributions of the entire population. This increase in total contributions generates the longevity dividend, which enriches society by a combination of economic benefits and social advancement.

The change in population structure – a one-time occurrence – proceeds rapidly during a limited time period before the structure stabilizes. If society does not take advantage of the years of the population shift, the opportunity to gain from the longevity dividend will be missed (Olshansky et al., 2016). Society retains the benefits gained through the longevity dividend and continues to develop, starting at the higher rate to the benefit of future generations. Societies can take advantage of this time-limited transition by making strategic choices to increase the longevity dividend.

What would be lost if this opportunity is missed? Can any country afford to forgo the value of the human capital of around a fifth of its population? The decision is about more than just fairness. It is about realizing the potential major national benefit which could give the country a one-time boost that will improve the lives of the current and future generations.

The duration of the population transition allows society to use the time and resources to adapt. It alters the public discussion from the burden of old age to the potential of the extra years of later life to benefit society. Adjusting to the realities of a longer life span by developing the economic and social strategies to differently organize work, family, caring and a life cycle culture would proceed over a period of years. The transformation to a lifelong learning system enables people of all ages throughout life to use knowledge to make the longevity dividend a reality. A natural consequence of a life course perspective would be a society for all ages, where the roles of different ages are considered developmentally but also collectively for their unique contributions to life and society. Critical investments in each cohort, while keeping the lifetime needs and gains in mind, achieves optimum human development for all, which leads to long term societal advantages. A society is more productive and efficient when every citizen contributes to the best of their ability throughout life for societal benefit.

Greater longevity is an amazing social achievement. If societies choose to take advantage of longer lives, aging would be mainstreamed and re-imagined, rather than devalued and marginalized. Asset-based thinking through life and compensatory strategies for individuals' disadvantages at any age would improve the opportunities and experiences for everyone. It would change the quality of the later years and modify how society views age, aging and older people. A long horizon, considering how a whole life might unfold, grants individuals the flexibility to invest in themselves, achieve their potential and be valued members of society throughout life. Societal organization of labour, markets, education, housing, health, long term care, social security, transport and technology would be designed to function over the lifetime without disadvantaging any phase of life. The guarantee of positive aging over the lifetime for every birth cohort would reinforce intergenerational solidarity. A society for all ages values life as it is lived at every age.

References

Arrow, K., Dasgupta, P., & Mumford, K. (2014). Health capital. In UNU-IHDP & UNEP (Ed.), *Inclusive wealth report 2014. Measuring progress toward sustainability* (pp. 123–136). Cambridge University Press.

Bourdieu, P. (1973). Cultural reproduction and social reproduction. In R. Brown (Ed.), *Knowledge, education and cultural change. Papers in the sociology of education* (pp. 71–113). Routledge.

Cutler, D. M., & Lleras-Muney, A. (2006, June). *Education and health: Evaluating theories and evidence* (Working Paper 12352). National Bureau of Economic Research. https://www.nber.org/papers/w12352

Davis, D. D. (1986). The uniqueness of human learning. *Medical Hypotheses, 21*(2), 153–164. https://doi.org/10.1016/0306-9877(86)90005-8

Grossman, I., Na, J., Varnum, M. E. W., Park, D. C., Kitayama, S., & Nisbett, R. E. (2010). Reasoning about social conflict improves into old age. *Proceedings of the National Academy of Sciences of the United States of America, 107*(16), 7246–7250. https://doi.org/10.1073/pnas.1001715107

Keeley, B. (2007). *Human capital: How what you know shapes your life*. OECD Publishing. https://doi.org/10.1787/9789264029095-en

OECD. (2016). *Skills matter: Further results from the survey of adult skills*. OECD Publishing. https://doi.org/10.1787/9789264258051-en

OECD & Centre for Educational Research and Innovation. (2007). *Understanding the social outcomes of learning*. https://www.oecd.org/education/ceri/understandingthesocialoutcomesoflearning.htm

Olshansky, S. J., Martin, G. M., & Kirkland, J. L. (2016). *Aging: The longevity dividend.* Cold Spring Harbor Laboratory Press.

Population Division. (2022a). *Life expectancy at birth* [Data portal]. United Nations. Retrieved 6 January 2023. https://population.un.org/dataportal/data/indicators/61/locations/900/start/1960/end/2022a/table/pivotbylocation

Population Division. (2022b). *World population prospects 2022: Summary of results (UN DESA/POP/2022/TR/NO.3).* United Nations. https://www.un.org/development/desa/pd/sites/www.un.org.development.desa.pd/files/wpp2022b_summary_of_results.pdf

Population Division. (2022c). *World population prospects: The 2022 revision* [Data portal]. United Nations. Retrieved 6 January 2023. https://population.un.org/dataportal/data/indicators/46/locations/900/start/1950/end/2100/table/pivotbyvariant

Sandel, M. J. (2020). *The tyranny of merit: What's become of the common good?* Farrar, Straus and Giroux.

Woolcock, M. (2001). The place of social capital in understanding social and economic outcomes. *ISUMA The Canadian Journal of Policy Research, 2*(1), 11–17.

Chapter 2
The Evolution of the Later Years of Life

2.1 Later Years of Life: An Evolving Life Phase

What a lifetime of difference a generation makes! In their long lives, people over 75 now run marathons, lead countries, fly into space and run businesses so it is no longer news. In developed countries a generation of individuals traditionally spans a period of about 25 years from a person's birth to the birth of the person's first child. Those in the same generation are characterized by their education, economic status and life style, which affect their response to societal roles, world events and technology. Enduring factors shape their lifetimes but changes are also occurring at a faster rate. This means there are not only differences between generations but also differences between cohorts born at the beginning of a generation and those born near the end. Each generation will make its own history. The alpha generation of individuals born between 2010 and 2024 is the first one to be immersed in smart technology their entire lives, experiencing interconnectivity and artificial intelligence. But for the generation of 75-year olds and over, smart technology arrived late in their lives. Longevity creates change in unanticipated ways.

Life expectancy has been growing at a rapid pace – an unforeseen human achievement resulting from increased survival rates of people around the world. For most of human history the average life expectancy at birth was only about 30 years. Now, global greying is a widespread phenomenon. The world average life expectancy in 2021 was 73 years and 2 months. In 1970 – just 50 years ago – it was about 58 years, and it now ranges between 80 and 85 years in developed countries (Population Division, 2022).

Greater longevity affects population growth in several ways, none of which have occurred before. First, the average lifespan of people around the world will increase, and people are likely to live longer than their parents. Life expectancy is by 2050 projected to exceed 80 years in 91 countries (Bloom, 2020). The average global life expectancy at 65 years of age will be 2 years longer in 2050 than it was in 2020

S. Brink, *The Longevity Dividend*, International Perspectives on Aging 39,
https://doi.org/10.1007/978-3-031-35335-2_2

(Population Division, 2019). The number of centenarians is projected to grow from about half a million today to almost 3.7 million in 2050 (Stepler, 2016). About 1 in 1000 centenarians live longer than 110 years to become super centenarians (Maier et al., 2010). Gerontology Wiki identified 62 validated super centenarians in the world in early 2023 (Oldest Living People, 2023).

Second, never before have so many people lived past 65 years of age. The population of persons aged 65–100 will grow rapidly during a time when the overall population growth is slowing. The world population grew by more than 2% per year in the late sixties and will grow at a quarter of that rate by 2050. The Population Division (2019) projects that the global population 65 and over may nonetheless more than double from 703 million in 2019 to 1.5 billion in 2050. It projects the percentage of the global population 65 and over to increase from 9% in 2019 to 16% in 2050. Almost one in six people will thus be aged 65 years and over in 2050. Proportions in individual countries will vary. Currently Japan has the highest population aged 65 and over at 28%, triple the world average. But by 2050, this proportion will be more common with over 29 countries having a greater percentage than Japan has today. Korea is projected to surpass Japan to record a historically unprecedented 38.1% of its population aged 65 and over (Bloom, 2020).

Third, life expectancy is at present greater in developed countries. But population aging has been fastest in Eastern and South Eastern Asia, where the percentage of the population aged 65 and over almost doubled from 6% to 11% between 1990 and 2019 (Population Division, 2019). Countries with populations that are aging the fastest have less time to adjust to their population changes. For instance, it took about 70 years for the United States to progress from an aging society to an 'aged society', but forecasted projections suggest that the same transition would only take about 20 years in Brazil and China (AARP, 2022). Countries that aged slowly without taking action to benefit from longer lives will only have little time remaining to take advantage of the potential gains.

Fourth, the older cohorts among the 65 and over population will grow faster than the younger ones. The growth of the population 75 years and over will proceed at a faster rate than the general population in the next two decades, particularly in developed countries.

As an example, in one projection Canada's population as a whole would grow at yearly rates calculated to average 0.9% from 2021 to 2050, affected by both fertility and immigration (Statistics Canada, 2022b). However, the older age groups would grow faster, averaging 2.2% per year, 4.0% and 4.7% for, respectively, the 75–84 age group, the 85–94 group and the 95 and over group. Figure 2.1 illustrates the effects of the differential rates of growth in 5-year age groups from 60 years and up from 2021 to 2050, showing particularly the increases in the oldest groups.

In just 30 years, the world will be peopled differently. Population aging and growing life expectancy will result in a new and larger segment of people over 75 years of age experiencing later life – a new life phase not widely experienced before. The unprecedented growth of the population segment of people 75 and over makes it important to develop a better understanding of this uncharted territory. This stage could last a fifth or more of people's lives in most developed countries and can

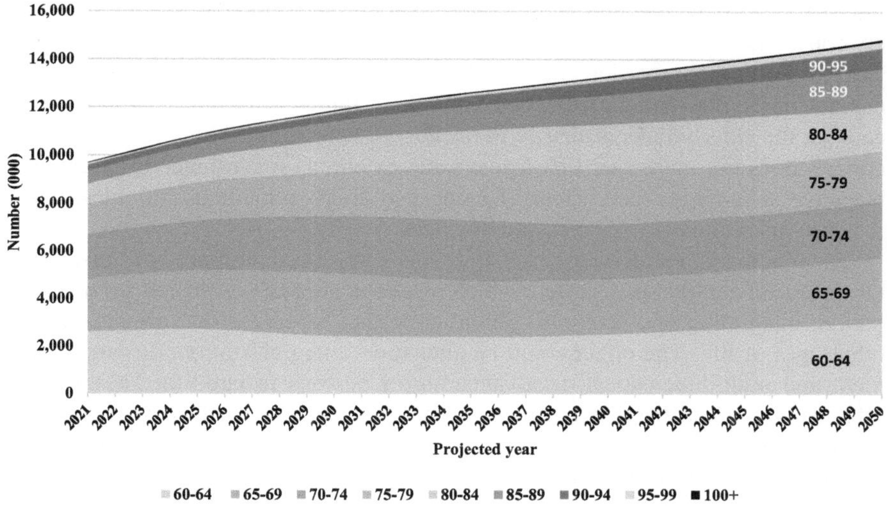

Fig. 2.1 Projected growth of Canadians 65 years to over 100 years shows faster growth of the older population, 2021–2050. (Data from Statistics Canada, 2022b, Table 17-10-0057, M4 medium-growth scenario)

extend for 25 years or more. As women live longer on average, women at these older ages predominate to an extent rarely seen in other age groups.

2.2 Aging in New Ways

The fast growth in both longevity and population aging has outpaced the advances that need to be made in understanding the changes in aging and the role of older people in society. The current concept of old age is captive to outdated legacy thinking. The paradigm freeze, where new future thinking or improvement do not occur despite the dissonances with reality, prevents the re-imagining of aging in society. Research on population aging has usefully explored how individuals and countries cope with longevity, such as the book titled The 100 Year Life: Living and Working in an Age of Longevity (Gratton & Scott, 2016). The Lee and Mason (2011) book focused on the implications of population aging for the macroeconomy, including economic growth, human capital, public finance and intergenerational equity. Further, country experiences show that social progress requires adaptations by both individuals and society.

There is a disconnect between the way older people experience their later years of life and the way society continues to view this stage. The tendency for society to envision old age as an unproductive short extension of adulthood has resulted in benign neglect, at best, or exposure to harsh exclusion from social, political and economic dimensions of society, at worst. This attitude has slowed progress and flavoured the social perception of the later years of life, which affects the way society considers the aging process and the role and status of people in this stage of life. There is far more discussion about the burden of the retired population measured as dependency ratios than there is about the role of falling birth rates. The concept of care for the elderly links primarily to the cost of health care, but care for other life cohorts does not make that link to the same extent, as for instance in infant care. Negative stereotypes feed a fear of aging and create prejudicial attitudes, which result in discriminatory policies and practices.

The tendency to undervalue later life makes the social contract omit this phase. Or the social contract is distorted, which results in later life exclusion from participation, integration and access to public and other resources that are available to other ages of life. The effect could be alienation, marginalization, disenfranchisement and multidimensional disadvantaging of persons in late-life. They may be effectively shunted from the mainstream and relegated to the fringe of society. It erodes the basic idea of a social contract that is fair for all generations and ensures that lives of citizens of any age have equal value. In the future, fairness across time should continue to benefit each generation as it ages into the next. The 50-plus population now represents four generations (up to Generation X, born between 1965 and 1980) and by 2031 it will include millennials. Generation Y (born between 1981 and 1996) will enter the 50-plus cohort in 2047, less than 25 years away. The first step for societal adaptation is to understand the characteristics of people in their later years of life. These characteristics could provide insights into how aging transpires over a longer life course.

2.3 Changing Life Course

The longer later life extends the life span and changes the life course. Traditionally, the preschool years were followed by a long period of education and preparation for the labour market and adulthood. Adult life was marked by a career, family and saving for retirement. Most pensions were designed for eligibility for retirement at age 65, followed by pension income for about 10 years. The growth in life expectancy has created disarray in this pattern. The prolongation of life is obvious, but the stages are no longer as discrete. Nor are the primary functions associated with each life stage as distinct as they were in the past. For example, lifelong learning opportunities have enabled people to gain university degrees after retirement. People divorce and marry late in life. Work can start early with studies still underway. In later life, work can be combined with retirement. Even preschool children use technology. Later life can have characteristics and activities of the earlier stages in addition to having those specific to the later years.

Studies on de-standardization of the life course have identified differences in the prevalence of life events, timing, spread and order. Changes in transition markers and linkages between them explain why the likelihood of identifying a standard pattern of biography is scant. There are also differences due to gender, socio-economic status, culture and country of residence (Widmer & Ritschard, 2009). Life courses have become individual and further affected by personal agency.

Chronological age is a poor predictor of health, life activities, experiences and skills. Such varied patterns result in very individual life courses. Standardized functional age, calculated as chronological age in combination with physiological, psychological, and social function, would be useful but is complicated and inaccurate because of the diversity of cohorts and the individuality of lives.

Gratton and Scott (2016), among others, suggest that the long arc of life will be split into multiple life stages, but it is not clear that the stages can be well defined. When stages are blurred and life activities are combined and displaced, policies targeted to age groups will not be efficient or effective. All-ages-thinking supplemented by life course policies based on need may be a strategy to ensure that rights and resources are equally available through life regardless of age.

The new life course is more than a sequence of preordained socially defined events lived over a longer period of time. In a traditional life course there were periods where some life roles were more concentrated than others. Middle age years were the peak career years, with high demands from family life, often accompanied by financial pressures arising from home mortgage payments, children's education costs and saving for retirement. It is becoming more common to organize the life course differently. There can be breaks in careers or sabbaticals, work beyond age 65, four-day work weeks with the same number of hours, time off for further education or maternity and paternity leave for child nurturing. Lives are constructed so that individuals can redistribute life roles without lowering pensionable service time and retirement income.

Intermittent influences create a seismic shift in each life course, both in early and late ages, compared to the traditional life path. The influence of societal change on the life course is intertwined with individual change (Caspi et al., 1989) and external factors such as technology developments. While the medical, social and cultural factors are shared, biological and personal agency and timing of decisions cause individual variations.

These factors have a strong role in changing the life course of individuals. The pace and specifics of the changes are uncertain, particularly in later life. Ambiguity can lead some societies to continue to characterize the older individuals as a population in physical and cognitive decline. They are perceived as low contributors because of their often unfairly attributed poor participation in society. However, the individuals in the older population are creating the years of later life that they desire.

2.3.1 A Later Life Phase of Two Decades or More

The United Nations has recognized three solid facts about population aging: It is unprecedented, is without parallel in human history and will be more rapid in the twenty-first century; it is a pervasive global phenomenon and countries that start aging later but age faster have less time to adjust; and it is enduring because it will not reverse itself to more youthful populations (Population Division, 2002). Population projections indicate that in developed countries a quarter of the population is over age 65 and this proportion is likely to grow. The disruption of the past trend means that the current aging population is at the cusp of momentous change in terms of numbers of older people and patterns of aging.

Two decades of later life will be the average. Later life will be as long as childhood and youth combined. Furthermore, the length of later life continues to increase due to improved life styles, diets, hygiene and exercise, despite a temporary dip due to the pandemic-related losses from 2020.

Current views of old age are already outdated. A future perspective can dramatically alter the calculus of longevity as more people live healthier lives. Anti-senescence researchers question what the limits of life are and seek to alter aging and prolong life. This could enable more people to live even longer, as described in the recent book Ageless (Steele, 2020). Anti-aging senolytic drugs can clean up aging cells and improve immunity to help people stay healthier longer in old age (Kyriazis, 2016). Extraordinary measures are not necessary because even simple interventions can make a difference to function. Although multi-sensory processing decline and aging of the brain are correlated, such age-related degeneration can be reduced or even eliminated (Leon & Woo, 2018). Researchers suggest that challenging people physically and cognitively by enriching their sensory environment (visual, auditory, food, etc.) could reverse poor cognitive functioning and further increase healthy longevity.

If life extends to a hundred years, later life will consume one quarter of the life span. Some of the ways in which changes are affecting the last decades of life are discussed below.

Working Years and Retirement

The retirement years are being redesigned to match the health and capabilities of older persons. The twenty or so extra years of later life does not mean a long-drawn-out old age but rather a differently experienced phase. There are indications of a structural lag (White Riley et al., 1994) in the form of an imbalance between the transformation in the aging process over the life course and the social structures that provide meaningful opportunities and reward people at various ages.

Traditionally adults worked for decades, often for a single enterprise, then retired at age 65 and lived on their pensions for a decade or so. However, with increasing longevity, the time in retirement can be as long as 25 years or more though there are national variations (Fig. 2.2). The OECD (2019a) estimates that in developed countries, men could expect to spend 17.9 years in retirement while women will spend 22.5 years on average. Women thus tend to spend almost five years more in retirement on average than men. Risks of poverty among women in retirement is increased in countries where there is low female employment, poor pension systems or high gender pay gaps.

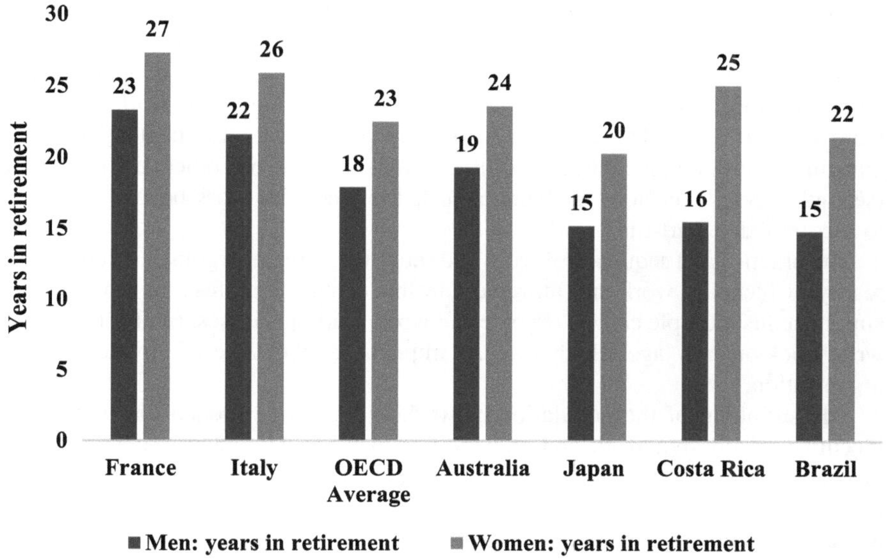

Fig. 2.2 Retirement can be as long as 25 years. Expected years in retirement in selected countries, 2017. (Data from OECD, 2019a, Figure 5.13)

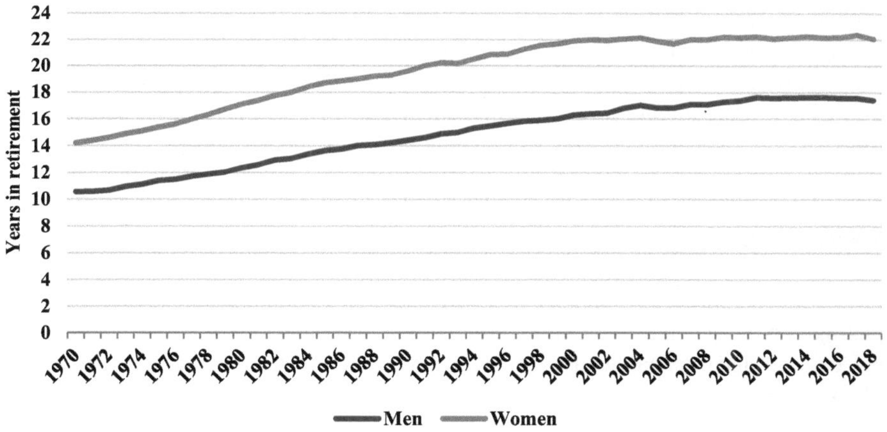

Fig. 2.3 Years in retirement for both men and women grew by about 8 years from 1970 to 2018 in the OECD area. (Data from OECD, 2019b, Figure 3.2)

The average number of retirement years has increased over time in most countries due to greater longevity. In 1970 men in OECD countries were retired for about ten years but by 2017, the time in retirement had increased to 18 years, as seen in Fig. 2.3 (OECD, 2019b). The increase was similar for women, with the years in retirement growing from fourteen years in 1970 to 22 years in 2017.

Age 65 is still considered a threshold for retirement and old age, but this is no longer universally valid in practice. Though eligibility for pensions often remains at age 65 or slightly older, many countries no longer have a mandatory age for retirement. In reality, older people have personalized ways of combining work and retirement over time. While some stretch out the process of retirement by working part-time, returning on contract, or filling in for staff on leave, others opt for encore (second) careers. Pensions are being adjusted to recognize work beyond age 65 or to accommodate part-time work.

The practice and sequence of work and retirement are undergoing evolution. The reality of blending work and retirement in this century manifests in sequential or simultaneous multiple careers. People can work, start businesses, run for office and write books at any age which was the impetus for the 'Age of No Retirement' organization.

The shrinking of the population of working age in developed countries is an incentive to redesign work and careers. For instance, Germany issued statistical projections showing that the number of people of working age would decline by between 1.6 and 4.8 million in the next 15 years (Statistisches Bundesamt, 2022). In addition, young people spend more years in education preparing for work and their careers, thereby further reducing the size of the workforce. If older people with high skills and human capital are unused, economies will forgo the benefit of this cognitive surplus. Expanding the economy requires employing and retaining older workers. The skills of older workers and their value to employers and corporations are not always recognized. They may have less formal education or may have graduated a long time ago, but they could have years of experience while they learned on the job during their careers. If they worked for one employer, they would be a repository of corporate memory. Since they are familiar with products and processes over the years of work, they are able to innovate products and processes.

Societal Expectations of Aging in Later Life

Ever since centuries ago Shakespeare wrote about second childhood in the famous passage on the seven ages of man, older people have been confirmed to be in physical decline and incapable of contributing to society. The negative stereotypes of older adults as frail, dependent, incompetent and helpless lead to ageism and an undesirable status in society (Bodner et al., 2018). Compassionate ageism is inexcusable since it expresses, in a subtly disempowering way, the acceptance of the stereotype of needy older adults as non-contributing members of society.

Efforts have been made to update ideas about life stages and to bring them closer to reality. One of the earliest works to describe a lifelong process in relation to the time was that of Erikson (1994) in the 1950s. In his 'Eight stages of man' he described, in a single life stage of old age over 65, the tension between integrity and despair: a sense of fulfillment from accomplishments in life diluted by regret for things still left undone. The contribution of these later years of life to society was also discussed. Erikson and Erikson (1998) described the concept of generativity, or the role in perpetuating culture and transmitting values to the next generation as custodians of culture. Older people's thoughts may turn to legacy in order to leave behind a desirable world to their children and grandchildren. They express wider concern for the well-being of future generations (Moody, 2008). The Gerotranscendence theory proposes that aging persons experience a cognitive transformation from a materialistic perspective towards a more cosmic oneness with the universe and a sense of connectedness with past and future generations (Tornstam, 1994). These theories are motivated by accepting the approach of the end of life rather than reimagining what a last quarter century of life could be.

Much of the thinking about aging was rooted in a time when life expectancy was shorter. The social construction of aging in real time entails an improved understanding of the prolonged life course and the role and status of people in later life. Such understanding would result in the creation of better fitting social norms in society as they relate to the aging of the population. This development has not yet been achieved, since outdated views of aging persist without keeping up with the growth of longevity.

2.4 An Evolving Life-Course Theory of Development Rather Than a Life-Stage Theory

Research on current life-course changes is enriching our knowledge on the later years, which could lead to a viable theory. In the past it was simpler to stratify society by age groups or life stages on the assumption that they would share not only similar experiences and culture but also similar needs for assistance or resources and status and roles relative to other groups (White Riley et al., 1972).

Currently evolving complexity derives from multiple new and disruptive factors. Though events, transitions and trajectories are recognized, they are still based on linear life stages and identical impacts on individuals. However, people of the same age in later life are now too dissimilar in experiences and transitions to form a homogeneous group. Elder Jr (1985) theorized that the life course is affected by five key principles of life style development: human agency, historical time, geographic place, timing of decisions and linked lives. The changes within a person's life span and the changes in contextual and historical time occur simultaneously and at different speeds, so their concurrent, lagged and reciprocal interactions are hard to comprehend. Each individual's life can be unique and the life stages no longer have predictable patterns of the roles and events expected by society. Not everyone will experience life events such as marriage and children, and the sequence of these events may be varied and non-traditional – from a heterosexual marriage to a homosexual one, for example. The theory would need to consider the diversity among people in later life. The tradition of life stages described by age-differentiated groups sharing the experience of social phenomena that vary little across time and place may have to be abandoned or drastically modified.

Developing a life-course theory that is meaningful in the twenty-first century is complex. That individual development is a lifelong process is instinctively understood, but the negative perceptions of aging prevent it from being accepted as continuing to the end of life. A realistic theory must integrate evolving knowledge about multiple pathways through life and take into account all the impacts experienced through a lifetime of aging (Haight et al., 2002). It should also recognize the potential of later life during which multidimensional societal contributions may be made.

2.5 Characteristics of People in Later Years of Life

Because they are associated with age group norms, traditional life stages are predictable in their characteristics in the life course. They are related to roles, status in society and social contributions. However, the concept of later life is not only new but is in flux. To describe it as leading to the end of life is inadequate. Furthermore, there is great diversity among individuals in the later life stage. Perhaps later life should simply be described as the last two decades of life for now.

2.5.1 Later Life Rather Than Old Age

In countries with long-lived residents, more babies born since 2000 will celebrate their 100th birthdays with less disability and fewer functional limitations if the present yearly growth in life expectancy continues (Christensen et al., 2009). Life expectancy is growing rapidly. With each passing year, the newly born live about three months longer on average than those born in the prior year (Easterbrook, 2014). Chronological age no longer serves as a valid proxy to describe the location on the trajectory of a person's life. Basically, it only indicates how long an individual has lived and perhaps the experiences and capacities that may be suggestive of that age. However, the extreme diversity in people's lives makes chronological age a poor predictor of their potential.

The challenge is to understand how the increase in human functionality evolves with the growth of longevity. Very early, Hersch (1948) recognized the mismatch and attempted to assess capacity based on 'potential life years'. More recently, countries rely on indicators such as average 'disability free years' for policy decisions. 'Prospective age' identifies people with the same expected remaining years of life and interprets patterns of survival (Sanderson & Scherbov, 2019). While these indicators recognize the possibility of more activity in later years, the use of averages hides the variability among people in this life stage.

2.5.2 *Family and Living Arrangements in Later Life*

Marriage was an expected life event for people born after World War II. In the United States, 91% of men and 92% of women aged 60–69 have been married, and the rate is 95% for men and women aged 70 and over (Gurrentz & Mayol-Garcia, 2021). These rates are much higher than for all men and all women aged 15 and over (63% and 69%, respectively).

Many people remain married in the later years of life. In Canada, a fifth of the age group of 85 years and over lived with a married spouse or common law partner. Fewer than about 5% of marriages last 50 years but, in the United States, a surprising number celebrate their golden anniversaries and beyond (United States Census Bureau, 2011). In the United States, among those 60–69 years, 46% of men and 39% of women are still married to the first and only person they married (Gurrentz & Mayol-Garcia, 2021).

The family cycle is changing swiftly, however. Unlike previous generations, people marry late or do not marry. Many developed countries have moved from high to lower fertility as couples have fewer children. The average age of parents when their first child is born in Canada is 30 years or older. Couples have no or only one or two children. Although grown children move out of the parental home, they may move back. In the past, child rearing was a major family role, followed by retirement and a slower pace of life, but this has changed. A couple may have additional years as 'empty nesters' to engage in fulfilling activities, travel and new social relationships.

As the stigma of divorce has faded, more people divorce in old age – silver or diamond splitters. The rates of remarriage or unions are higher among men than women. In 2012 in the United Kingdom, the number of grooms and brides in their late sixties increased by 25% and 21%, respectively, from 2011. One in ten had been single, two thirds were divorced and the rest widowed (Roberts, 2014).

The traditional nuclear family is now just one among other family forms. Baby boomers made cohabiting more socially acceptable, often as a prelude to marriage. Cohabiting and also raising children together is now more common than before. Baby boomers now in their later years are making non-cohabiting unions more acceptable as well. Many form lasting relationships but choose not to marry because of potentially complicated relationships with their children and difficulties with the management of financial assets (Cheng, 2019).

Adults who had children are empty nesters in later life, but if their children and grandchildren reside in their area, they can maintain close relationships. During the Covid pandemic from 2020, many grandparents were willing and able to provide grandchild care and home-schooling services while their children worked away from or at home.

Relationships between living family members are being redefined as the oldest members of the family may live to see their great-great-grandchild. The grandparenting role has grown in importance, and grandparents may have a relationship with their grandchildren until their teenage years. Four and five generations of the same family may be alive at the same time. Children may have only a single sibling and fewer cousins in their own generation than members in earlier generations had.

Some decisions regarding residential options are predominantly associated with people in later life. The first is to downsize from the family home to a smaller dwelling, perhaps in the same or nearby familiar community but without the need to be responsible for yard work and home maintenance. The second is to move to a retirement community, inhabited by people of similar age. Some move permanently while others live there part of the time. Such homes may even be located in another country. The living space may be barrier-free and the community offers activities and services that cater to people in this life stage. The third is a move out of the family home and to a much smaller space in a care home, where food, housekeeping and health services and care are provided. Nonetheless, the vast majority of people in later life live with their spouse or alone in their own home according to their preference (Sinha, 2020).

Residential decisions will depend on individual factors such as health, disabilities, finances and potential support from family and friends. They will also depend on policy factors such as pensions, housing subsidies, community home care possibilities and health care. For example, in Sweden and Denmark only 5% of older people live with their children, while in southern European countries, such as Spain, Greece and Italy, about a third of older people live with their children (Ogg & Renaut, 2006).

Autonomy is often associated with living independently in one's own home. Klinenberg (2012) suggests the appeal of continuing to live alone is a social experiment at odds with past human history. It may have arisen from the influence of a number of social factors, such as the cult of the individual and the improved social status of women. There are risks involved in the choice to maintain an independent home, such as spousal abuse among couples or loneliness if a person lives alone.

The loss of a spouse is a common experience for people in later life. About 25% of adults in later life live alone in Canada as either unmarried, divorced or widowed persons (Tang et al., 2019). The number of people over sixty-five living alone is relatively high in other western countries, such as 38.4% in France, 32.7% in England and Wales and 30.8% in the United States (Reher & Requena, 2018). The rate of living alone rises with age as the urge to live independently can be strong despite the loss of spouse due to death or divorce. In Sweden, 41% of people aged 65 and over lived alone in 1975 (Sundström et al., 2002). In 2000, 58% of people aged 75 and over lived alone when this situation had become more common. In Canada, living alone increases with later life age as seen in Fig. 2.4. This is the case especially for women who generally outlive their spouses. The pattern of more women in later life living alone is seen in Europe as well. The share of women 65 and over living alone in 2018 in the European Union was 40.2% while the corresponding share for men was 21.8% (Eurostat, 2020).

In Canada, over half of those 85 and over still live in their single-family homes. Over half of women and 27% of men aged 85 and over live alone and rely on support of friends and relatives (Tang et al., 2019). In 2009, 53% of people aged 85 and over lived in a single-family home, compared with 71% aged 75–84, 70% aged

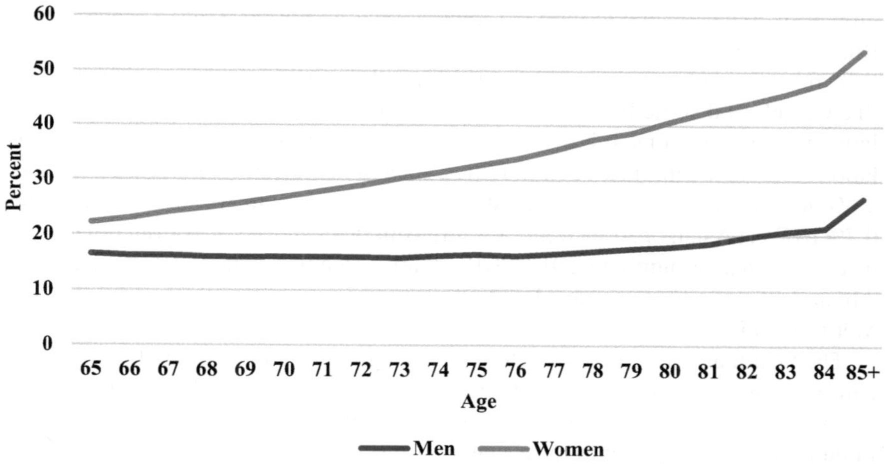

Fig. 2.4 More women than men live alone in old age, Canada, 2016. Percent of population, by age and sex, living alone. (Data from Tang et al., 2019, Chart 4, Data table)

65–74 and 75% aged 55–64 (Turcotte, 2012). People's access to services may be uneven because of factors such as insufficient supply in rural areas or limited affordability. Underutilization of large homes in which older people live is noted in many countries, while younger families are unable to find large enough homes. In 2018, 47% of people aged 65 and over lived in underoccupied homes in the European Union, compared to 31% of people aged 18–64 years (Eurostat, 2020).

Collective dwellings are chosen because of advanced age or disabling conditions, such as dementia or high need for services. In Canada, 28% of people aged 85 and over lived in collective dwellings such as nursing homes and residences for older people in 2016 (Statistics Canada, 2022a). This proportion grew to 54% among those 100 years and older.

2.5.3 Diversity in the Later Years of Life

People in the later years of life are heterogeneous and diverse. During their long lives, they have had different educational achievements, work careers, socio-economic outcomes, social mobility, life experiences and social networks.

Moreover, the composition of older people in the later years of life within a country is dynamic, due to different rates of immigration, fertility and mortality. For instance, in the United States, though the population continues to grow, the non-Hispanic White-alone population is projected to shrink over the coming decades from 199 million in 2020 to 179 million in 2060. The Two or More Races population is projected to be the fastest growing over the next several decades, followed by single-race Asians and Hispanics of any race. Unlike the other groups, the high growth of Asians is due to high net international migration (United States Census Bureau, 2019).

A mix of people of many nationalities and ethnic origins is observed in countries like Canada and some European Union countries with a high immigration rate and indigenous populations. It is also observed where there is a high foreign older population residing in retirement communities, such as in Florida or Gibraltar. In Canada, 4.6% identified as East or Southeast Asian, 3.1% as South Asian, 1.3% as Black, 0.7% as West Asian or Arab, 0.3% as Latin American and 2.3% as from other ethnic or cultural backgrounds in 2017–2018 (Public Health Agency of Canada, 2020). About 1.9% of older people identified as Indigenous, specifically First Nations, Métis or Inuit.

The health and longevity of heterogeneous groups can be affected by particular cultural influences, both dietary choices and other health related behaviour. Cultural differences may be indicated by language differences. For example, in bilingual Finland, the life expectancy of a newborn girl with Swedish speaking parents is projected to be 85.7 years while it is 84.8 years for a newborn girl with Finnish speaking parents. For children of parents speaking both languages, there is an advantage if the child's first language is Swedish. The projected life expectancy of boys displays the same pattern (Reini & Saarela, 2021).

Stereotypes are not valid, so it is unfortunate that they nevertheless are often applied indiscriminately to all persons in the later years of life. Rather, society should value these older people's wide and varied experiences and acknowledge their continued contributions to society. With their variety of early experiences, ethnic and national backgrounds and spoken languages, these individuals contribute in different ways to society in their later years. They also enrich the national culture with arts and language from their personal experiences.

2.5.4 Health and Autonomy

People live longer and are healthier in their later years, compared to earlier generations (Healthy Aging and Wellness Working Group, 2006). The understanding of good health is undergoing a change, and it is no longer about peak performance or the total absence of disease. From a life course perspective, lifelong healthy aging is a combination of outcomes: adequate physical and mental wellness, satisfying social relationships, successful transitions leading to continued quality of life and ability to act on life opportunities. From lived experience, most older people consider good health as a condition that fosters high physical and mental functioning, independence, security, social engagement and normal daily life.

People live longer and with fewer disabilities than the generations before them. While the prevalence of chronic conditions and disabilities increases with age, a life course approach to prevention and treatment would yield benefits. For instance, among individuals in Canada aged 15–24 years, 13% had a disability, but among those aged 75 years and over the rate rose to 47% (Morris et al., 2018). The majority of Canadians in later life do not have disabilities, although multimorbidity or multiple disabilities increase with age (Table 2.1). Many older persons reported a high level of functioning and autonomy, since their disabling conditions are mild and can be managed with treatment, prosthesis or environmental modifications so that they do not hamper active aging.

The leading causes of 'years lived with disability' among people 65 and over in Canada were chronic conditions such as diabetes, high systolic blood pressure, stroke, heart failure and chronic obstructive pulmonary disease (Public Health Agency of Canada, 2020). The years lived with disability rises sharply with age for Alzheimer's disease and other dementias as well as cardiovascular diseases. However, a large proportion of older people are able to live active satisfying lives.

Quality of life and risk of poor health are also affected by health habits such as poor nutrition and lack of exercise, which can result in underweight or overweight. Based on their body mass index (BMI) about 30% of older Canadians were at normal weight, while about 40% were overweight and 28% were obese (Public Health Agency of Canada, 2020).

The prevalence of most chronic diseases increases with age and over time. In Canada, among those aged 85 years and over, the diseases with the highest prevalence were hypertension (83%), osteoarthritis (54%), ischemic heart disease (42%), osteoporosis (37%) and chronic obstructive pulmonary disease (27%) (Public Health Agency of Canada, 2020). It is estimated that 37% of older persons have at least two chronic diseases, and more women than men 85 years and over have multimorbidity. Dutch research found that chronic disease or multimorbidity affect older men and women differently, which affects the number of years that they live with the effects. For example, men spent more years living with coronary heart disease (7.6 years at age 65 and 3.7 years at age 85) while more Dutch women coped with osteoarthritis (11.7 years at age 65 and 4.8 years at age 85) (Botes et al., 2018).

Lifestyle behaviour also affects chronic diseases. Three in particular – smoking, harmful use of alcohol and inactivity – have been related to chronic diseases. Smoking is associated with lung disease, cancer and heart disease. About 9% of people 65 and over smoke in the United States and Canada (United Health Foundation, 2022; Statistics Canada, 2022c). Alcohol abuse is linked with osteoporosis, diabetes, high blood pressure, and stroke. Physical activity can delay, prevent or manage many chronic diseases, in addition to maintaining muscle tone and a

Table 2.1 Disabilities among Canadians in later life, 2017

Condition	65–74 years (%)	75 years and older (%)
Without disabilities	68.0	52.6
With disabilities	32.0	47.4
One disability type	23.3	19.8
Two or three disability types	41.6	35.9
Four or more disability types	35.1	44.2

Source: Morris et al. (2018, Chart 2)

sense of healthy wellbeing. Inactivity has been associated with age and also with gender, since women are significantly more likely to be inactive. In the United States, 26.9% of adults aged 65–74 years and 35.3% of adults aged over 75 years were inactive (Watson et al., 2016).

Research has identified differences between objective and subjective measures of aging, where older people may not meet the objective criteria for successful aging but a majority would meet the subjective criteria. Only 15% of older people met the criterion of 'absence of diseases', but 84% and 90% met the criteria, respectively, of 'life satisfaction' and 'self-rated successful aging' (Jeste et al., 2010). Though a person in later life may have chronic conditions or disabilities, most persons experience 'good' health as long as they can manage their health situations while continuing their daily activities and interests. In 2017–2018, almost half of Canadian older people perceived their health as very good or excellent, and over 72% thought their mental health was very good or excellent regardless of chronic conditions or minor disabilities (Public Health Agency of Canada, 2020).

Health is more and more seen as a positive resource for everyday living as experienced by people as they age. Chronological age can be a poor predictor of wellness and also of declines that are associated with aging. Research has indicated that a privileged, active 70-year-old man with a healthy weight can have the cardiovascular capacity of an inactive, overweight man who is 10–15 years younger (Shephard, 1998).

Consideration of health in later years is still hampered by outdated thinking about aging as a period of decline. Geriatrics is a challenging profession since about half of those 75 years and over are in good health without disabilities and need to maintain their health, while many others need major interventions and care. Health care systems tend to focus on treatment rather than health promotion and disease prevention. Redirecting attention to the latter is required so that older people can maintain optimal health and quality of life. Preventive life course care can increase the numbers of people in good health in their later years.

2.5.5 Cognitive Abilities in Later Life

The distribution of cognitive abilities among people in the later life stage is very large, from those capable of amazing memory (mnemonic) tasks such as reciting a whole play by Shakespeare to those incapacitated with Alzheimer's disease. Cognitive abilities wane somewhat with normal aging, but most people in the later life stage continue their lives unhampered. The reduction in abilities is normal, similar to reduction in physical abilities which is accepted as normal, such as not being able to hit a golf ball as far as a decade previously.

Brain functions are complex. At every age, people become better at some functions, remain stable at some and become worse at others. It is unlikely that one single age exhibits peak performance in all brain functions. Pragmatic intelligence and knowledge acquired through culture and experience generally remain stable through life. However, crystallized intelligence or accumulated knowledge and facts about the world tends to peak late in life, so while people in later life may be slower, they are more accurate and knowledgeable. Their emotional intelligence remains active and they are better able to relate to the emotional states of others (Hartshorne & Germine, 2015). Older adults often perform as well as or better than young adults on general knowledge (semantic memory) or vocabulary (lexical memory). But there is great heterogeneity.

Though aging causes some mental processes to proceed less quickly, this is not a disability or a disease. Cognitive aging does not involve neuro-degeneration or significant damage to the neurons or the brain structure. Not being able to remember a name or a word is a common experience. Metacognition, a part of cognition, creates the 'tip of the tongue' state because the item that cannot be retrieved is probably still stored in memory and, with more time and effort, it can be found. Older adults are good at retaining information but they may occasionally take longer to retrieve it. A typical 20-year-old may experience a 'tip of the tongue' state (lethologica) perhaps once a week, but by 70 years it could rise to about once a day (Seabrook, 2008).

The brain is a vital organ with unique characteristics. Neuroplasticity, or the normal brain's ability to modify its cells and synapse connections in response to demands encountered, continues through life. The brain also exhibits neuro-resilience, or the ability to repair and cope with damage while still functioning adequately, a characteristic called brain reserve. Histological evidence of damage repair has been found. Cognitive reserve is the capacity of the brain to optimize or maximize performance through recruiting different networks and alternate strategies. Brain scans have shown that, while youth tended to use the right hemisphere alone for a memory tasks, older people use both sides, indicating positive compensatory adaption (Hartshorne & Germine, 2015).

Moreover, brain processes can be supported by personal effort. Physical exercise increases growth factors which stimulate new neuronal connections between a number of important cortical areas of the brain (Molteni et al., 2004). Stimulating the brain through curious inquiry, engagement, learning and social interaction also increases neurogeneration.

Unfortunately, any cognitive decline in the later life stage is popularly linked with Alzheimer's disease or other dementia. Neither condition is part of normal aging. The risk of dementia and its prevalence are related to age. While only 2.2% of people aged 65–69 years have dementia, the numbers rise to 20.1% by age 85–89 years (Lim et al., 2016). The stereotype has resulted in the idea that in later life substantial societal participation is impossible for most people, despite successful careers by many in their eighties and nineties in politics, science and art, which has shown otherwise. It is a tremendous waste to forgo the societal contributions of the large number of people in later life.

Much research focuses on the growth in numbers of people with dementia, partly due to increasing longevity and growth in the older population. However, the incidence of dementia in Europe and North America declined by 13% per decade over the past 25 years consistently across studies (Wolters et al., 2020). In 2022, people with dementia numbered about 55 million globally, and this number is expected to rise to 78 million in 2030 (World Health Organization [WHO], 2022). By 2050, 153 million people are expected to be living with dementia worldwide, up from about 57 million in 2019 (GBD 2019 Dementia Forecasting Collaborators, 2022). Increases in obesity, cardiovascular disease, excessive alcohol consumption and diabetes will cause preventable dementia to increase in high income countries (Schwarzinger & Dufouil, 2022).

In sum, a large proportion of the population is healthy and active in later life. Even persons with chronic illness or disability function well in daily life and are able to participate in society. With more learning and better preventive care, the share of people in later life who are active is likely to rise.

2.6 Adapting Society to Later Life

Confronted with reality, society not only expects people in later life to adapt to contemporary society and its demands, but it also has to adapt to a population where a large segment of the population is independently active through the later years of life. Society will need to make systemic adaptations in regulations, environments, products and services. Intergenerational relationships will also change to meet the needs of all groups.

For illustrative purposes, a few selected areas of adaptation are discussed below.

2.6.1 Driving in the Later Years

The ability to drive a car is a major component of independence in many countries. Only about 40% of persons 75 years and over used public transport in Canada (Turcotte, 2012). Older people are generally safe drivers compared to some other age groups, since they often reduce risk of injury by wearing seat belts, observing speed limits and not drinking and driving. They drive less after dark, during rush hour or in bad weather, and avoid difficult roads such as high-speed highways and interchanges. Most trips are for essential errands, such as to the grocery, pharmacy or government service points. However, they are involved in traffic accidents at higher rate than the middle age group, but at a rate lower than young drivers.

In Canada in 2009, three-quarters (3.25 million) of people aged 65 and over had a driver‘s license. Of that number, about 200,000 were aged 85 and over (Turcotte, 2012). Since people in their Eighties and over are, and will continue to be, a fast-growing segment of the senior population, society has to expect the number of older drivers to increase at a rapid pace. There are parallels in other countries. The number of licensed drivers aged 65 and older in the United States increased by 68% from 2000 to reach more than 48 million in 2020 (Office of Highway Policy Information, 2018). This means that one out of every five drivers on US roads is in this age group. The motor vehicle death rate per 100,000 people among those 65 and over actually declined from 22.4 in 1999 to 15.5 in 2018, a 31% drop (George & Choi, 2022). By 2030, when 70 million Americans will be aged 65 and over, 85–90% are expected to drive (American Automobile Association, n.d.). In Europe, older drivers over age 65 are expected to become a quarter of all drivers on the roads in 2030 (SilverEco, 2018). There were 5.3 million Britons over 70 years with full driving license in 2018, among whom were more than 100,000 licensed drivers 90–99 years old (BBC News, 2019).

Societal adaptations could include improved licensing procedures and regulations, car design such as bumper cameras, and traffic flow engineering, down to road signs and street lighting. The potential of new technological innovations such as self-driving cars are discussed in a later section.

2.6.2 *The Reciprocal Impact of Technology and the Evolving Stage of the Later Years*

Growth in longevity affects the relationship a population has with technology. Technology is created at a speed greater than the rate of growth of longevity. This results in older generations having to adapt to new technologies as adults, while children are socialized with it in daily life. Differences in adapting to technology may be greater between generations that differ greatly in age than between adjacent generations. The oldest generations may thus be the most disadvantaged in this respect.

Technology development itself may also be affected if it proceeds without understanding that a major proportion of the population is growing older. Understanding this opens opportunities to serve the aging but growing market. It is unclear, however, how lucrative offering products and services to this market may be, compared to serving a market of the entire population the way telephone, radio and television became household products.

2.6.3 *Technology Use in the Later Years*

The pandemic years from 2020 showed that digital technology is a necessity – not an option – for participation in the economy and in society. Many basic activities of living and participating in society require the use of digital gadgets and the internet. The use of digital devices may become more universal after the pandemic speeded up penetration, utility and internet coverage.

Currently, the use of digital technology in the later years is mixed. Age matters but the factors that affect technology decisions for this age group are digital experience, technological familiarity, cost, personal utility, context and benefits. Although older people are said to shun technology, they rather tend to use it on their own terms. The pandemic gave an impetus for many of those staying at home to start using or to make greater use of technology with the help of family and caregivers. In the United States ownership of digital devices among people in their seventies is lower than those in their sixties, but the gap varies according to device (Table 2.2). Smart phones and tablets were popular devices.

The proportion of Canadians aged 65 and older who owned a smartphone increased from 58% in 2019 to 65% in 2020 (AGE-WELL Network of Centres of Excellence [NCE], 2020). Most of those who owned one (83%) used it daily. The proportion of Canadians aged 65 and older who used video-calling on their smartphones doubled between 2019 and 2020 to 23%. Already 72% of Canadians aged 65 and over felt confident using current technology. Nineteen percent of them shopped online for essential items such as groceries or used a variety of apps to access services, contacts and information. In the United States, 61% of people aged 65 and over owned a smartphone in 2021, compared to 96% of those aged 18–29 (Faverio, 2022). Seventy-five percent of those 65 and over were internet users. Americans aged 60 and over spent more than half their daily leisure time (just over four hours) at their TVs, computers, tablets or other electronic devices (Smith, 2014). Screen time has increased for those in their 60s, 70s, 80s and beyond, and with no difference between genders and education levels (Livingston, 2019). They use apps such as Medisafe to manage medications and Google maps to note their parking location. For those aged 55–75, daily use of smart watches reached 75%, higher than the younger generations (Deloitte, 2017). But many of those who were on the internet did not use social networking sites, and 56% said they would need help to connect with friends and family (Smith, 2014). Digital proximity was a poor substitute for social relationships for people in their later life years as shown during the pandemic. Cost for purchase and operation is also an issue for lower income older people.

The picture is different in other countries, however. In the European Union, 87% of people aged 75 and over had never been online (No Isolation, 2018). In Norway, the share of people in the 61–100-year category who did not use the internet fell from about 20% to about 10% between 2014 and 2018 (Slettemeås et al., 2018). In Japan, only 19% of people aged eighty and over owned a smart phone. In Japan, internet use declined sharply with age. For instance, 60% of those 70–79 years used the internet, but only 26% of those over 80 years did (Aung et al., 2022).

Table 2.2 Device ownership among US adults aged 60–69 and 70 years and older

Device owned (2019–2021)	60–69 years (%)	70 years and older (%)
Smart phone	88	72
Tablet	60	56
Smart TV	72	57
Home assistant	36	28
Wearables	33	21
Smart home technology	26	21

Source: AARP Research (2021, p. 18)

2.6.4 Working Remotely Through Technology

Not every person in their later years is employable or wants to work, but a growing number of older people continue to work for personal satisfaction, professional growth or needed income. The pandemic years have shown that, with technology, work locations can be changed, tasks can be reorganized and work time can be distributed in different ways. Technology has made working from home a reality, which expands the options for those older people who do not want to or cannot drive and which also makes self-employment and part-time work more feasible. The number of people who will want to work after 65 years of age is likely to grow, at the same time as the prime age labour force is likely to shrink. However, employability of older people will depend not only on their expertise and experience but also on their digital knowledge and skills. Attitudes towards older workers in the work place will also affect the growth in employability.

2.6.5 Factors That Will Affect Use of Future Technology in Later Life

Some key factors need to be considered for older persons to gain the maximum benefit from technology, whether common to all technologies or specific to technologies that target older consumers. Technology developments that positively affect the aging experience can be 'assistive' or particularly designed for an older user. In either case, technology design has to recognize that this population segment is very diverse. The growing but untapped potential market of willing older consumers is predictable and large. This can be the impetus for development since there is little risk in undertaking inclusive design. For example, Samsung announced a greater engagement with inclusive design (WARC, 2020). Regulations and standards regarding inclusive design (or universal design) can shape responses to market demand.

Inclusive design is the creation of mainstream products and services that are accessible to and usable by as many people as reasonably possible without the need for customized design or special adaptation (British Standards Institution, 2005). Inclusive design thus targets the widest range of capacities and competencies among the public, regardless of age. Rather than design for an average user, inclusive design accommodates as much of the consumer population as possible. For long term population-wide sales, any product which uses chips or software with inclusive design will be marketable, whether designed for the general public or for older consumers.

Accessibility, usability and affordability are the criteria most pertinent for later life among the criteria for inclusive design. Design options and testing should address the following conditions that are common among older people:

Visual: Visual impairments, macular degeneration and lack of visual clarity make reading small print on small telephone screens a challenge. Colour vision also diminishes with age, so the use of colour in user guides may be difficult for older users. High contrast, large screen, font magnification and less flickering of text and images can be helpful.

Auditory: Hearing impairments cause difficulties with sound notifications and alerts at higher frequencies.

Sensory: Cognitive dissonance due to the slight lag in video and audio component of online meeting and event platforms.

Ease of use: Applications and software must be simple and intuitive for use by older consumers, especially if they are not avid users of technology or if they are first time users. Voice control is easiest to use. Jargon and dense writing of security, privacy and user information are not helpful.

Response time: Variations in reaction and response time, particularly with scrolling text and sub- titles. Older people may also have reduced reactivity, making it difficult to respond to notifications within set times.

Reading and writing difficulties: Text to speech and speech to text can be made a standard choice. US statistics show that 23% of older adults find reading difficult or challenging (Smith, 2014).

Hand and finger mobility: Flexibility and fine motor skills are reduced with arthritis. Keying, especially typing with thumbs, can be difficult for people who do not have mobility in the first and second finger joints. Hand-eye co-ordination may be difficult on small devices, which is why some older users like tablets better than smart phones. Finger swiping is not a natural motion unless technology was introduced when young. Touch screens can be helpful.

To ensure ease of use and positive interaction with the products, assessing usability and consumer reactions will be valuable before they are marketed. Consumer testing should cover people of all ages and both genders and incorporate both inclusiveness criteria and the time needed to learn and complete tasks correctly and efficiently.

2.7 Technology Adoption in Later Life

Typically, early adopters are young and technologically savvy. However, market share is gained only when there is widespread penetration in the population, including the growing segment of people in the later years of life. Adoption among older consumers can be speeded up with inclusive strategies.

Many people in their later years have not grown up with technology or used technology at work. It is a new way of thinking and working for them, and they find it arduous and time consuming to learn to use the digital gadgets by 'playing' with the gadget and by trial and error. The earlier they start to use technology, the more comfortable they are. The older the novice, the less likely the person is to embrace the internet, social media, or smartphones (Hitlin, 2018). Most aging persons are not yet in the market for virtual reality or robotic care assistants.

A serious issue arises when technology is specifically developed for the older person but he or she is not able to use it without help. The need for its use and the benefits must be indisputable for them to embrace the technology. Simple ways to use it, such as a touch screen rather than complex key strokes may appeal to them. Text to voice and voice to text are also helpful as a standard feature on apps and as an option on information sites.

The potential benefits of technology adoption are considerable if it contributes to higher quality of life, greater convenience and efficiency and lower costs. The costs faced by older persons will depend on the size of the potential market and the universality of the product. Products specially designed for a limited market of older or disabled people may be more expensive to purchase and operate.

Adoption of technology can also have considerable negative dimensions for people later in life. They may be marginalized in the market by designs that exclude them, perhaps because consumer studies did not include them. They may need more assistance to learn how to operate digital health monitoring systems or security applications. In the area of cybersecurity, older people are frequent target of scams and frauds resulting in losses of both savings and privacy. Inequities among groups of people in later life in terms of health and quality of life may be exacerbated. This could result from those with higher incomes and better education being better positioned to acquire and learn modern technologies.

2.7.1 Technology Concerns of People 75 and Over

People who are not technologically adept or those who are new users of digital services are often the victims of hackers, who gain control of identities, entry into homes and vehicles as well as computers and bank accounts. Concerns about being defrauded and losing their security and privacy are common among technology users in later life. They are reluctant to put personal information or financial information on a computer, pay with a bank card or engage in internet banking. Increasing their internet security by frequently adjusting privacy settings and using long and complicated passwords for each app is not ideal for this age group. The privacy statements of many establishments are long and difficult to understand. Instructions using jargon in the name of legal precision are not clear for novice users. Products with software are unlike traditional mechanical products. Successive updates to phones, apps and laptops to improve security and add features are a new idea to people used to buying a product that remains stable. Users need to adopt a particular mindset to ensure updates are downloaded and to relearn operations or adapt practices for proper use. Technical support using language and didactics that are easily accessible for the novice consumer may be lacking. Video guidance showing step by step actions can be helpful, even if the process seems obvious to an experienced user.

Older people may resist making a large investment in money or time in a technically advanced product if they are unsure of having the skills to use it. Payment plans involving monthly payments for a product or service, similar to subscriptions, may be viewed negatively.

2.7.2 *Access to the Internet*

It is clear that internet use among persons 65 and over is increasing and the large use gap with younger generations is declining. The age gradient depends on characteristics such as education, health status and living arrangements. However, even when people in the older cohort have access to the internet, their connections often lack in reliability, strength, bandwidth or speed. This is a particularly common problem in rural and remote communities.

A country-wide reliable and strong internet availability can today be regarded as infrastructure as essential as roads. The Universal Declaration of Human Rights of the United Nations includes since 2016 wording in Article 19 that many interpret as access to and use of the internet being a human right. Access is especially important for older people to use services such as communication, telehealth and security services. Access, whether subsidized or not, needs to be affordable also for those older persons who are financially disadvantaged.

2.7.3 *Future Technology Which Will Benefit Consumers in Their Later Years*

There is promise but also hype about how future technology can encourage active lifestyles for people in their eighth, ninth and tenth decades. The hope is that technology can improve the capacity for self-care, ensure independence in homes, increase access to information, substitute for human services, compensate for diminished capacities or even disabilities and increase access to top quality services, products and care from anywhere in the world. One example of such ideas reaching high government levels was the report presented in 2016 to the president of the United States. It discussed, among other things, the use of personal robots, wearable devices for monitoring and telehealth, 'smart' homes, internet of things, autonomous vehicles and artificial intelligence (President's Council of Advisors on Science and Technology, 2016). A report in the United Kingdom considered the policy implications of several similar technological advancements in relation to the future of an aging population (Government Office for Science, 2016).

From the perspective of the later years in life, wider use of currently emerging technologies could make a vast difference. A sample of them are discussed below.

Technology assisted medical advances and telehealth: Telehealth includes technologies that improve health outcomes of older people by increased monitoring, such as measuring blood pressure, and improve sophisticated use of health data for diagnosis and individualized clinical treatment. Telehealth also includes providing remote health care. Better medical outcomes may result from digital processes, such as personalized 3D printed joints. Some technologies are evolving rapidly and need to be evaluated in terms of the benefits and cost savings in the immediate and medium term. People in later life are able to consult medical information, get second opinions and research treatment options to make wiser medical decisions. Other developments such as transplants of laboratory-created organs, therapeutic robotics, computer aided prosthetics and genomics may still be years away. The adoption of such technologies depends, on the one hand, on client acceptance and, on the other, on how quickly aging people, service users, professionals and carers are able and willing to use these technologies.

Transport: Public transportation, whether by rail, buses, taxis, ride sharing or others, are being redesigned to enable wider usage by a greater range of people. Barrier free access is now required by law in many places.

Some technological developments are making a difference by prolonging the driving years of older people while increasing the safety and comfort of all drivers. Examples are features such as rear-view cameras for backing and reversing, blind-spot warning systems and auto-parking technology.

The next generation of more autonomous vehicles could potentially increase older people's use of personal transportation without jeopardizing the safety of other road users. This would allow greater independence and social interaction.

Smart homes: A smart home is a residence that uses internet connected applications and devices to manage home systems, such as security, lighting and heating, and to possibly monitor and operate them remotely. Embedding chips and sensors in products and services can improve their processing, machine learning and intercommunication capabilities.

The key features and abilities of smart home technology are likely to include automation (incorporating automatic devices and performing automatic functions), multifunctionality (performing various tasks and generating various outcomes), adaptability (simultaneously adjusting to meet the different personal needs of resident users), interactivity (interacting among users and related products), and efficiency (performing functions that are time and cost saving as well as convenient).

While many elements of a smart home setup may be designed to facilitate the activities of households with children, there is also potential for them to support aging in place. Smart home technology can automate routine home tasks, medicine cabinets can check if daily doses of prescription medicine are taken and toilets sensors can monitor for signs of ill health by scanning waste (Austin, 2019). More than 20% of US people 60 years and over owned a device in the category smart home technology in 2019–2021 (Table 2.2).

2.8 Citizenship and Participation in Society in the Later Years

The understanding of what is involved in active citizenship and societal participation developed long before life expectancy significantly rose. There is consequently a tendency currently to continue to assume that people in their later years would be unable be involved in society. As a result, the role of people in this age group is often ignored.

Citizenship involves rights and responsibilities throughout life, regardless of age. The UN Universal Declaration of Human Rights from 1948, states that "All human beings are born free and equal in dignity and rights" (United Nations, 1948). This is the basis for ensuring economic, social, political, cultural and civic rights for all to ensure a life free from want and fear. However, people did not live as long in 1948 as they do in this century. While the declaration does not specifically protect against age discrimination, some national laws provide a legal framework for older people to have equal status in law and access to public policy and resources. For example, the Canadian Charter of Rights and Freedoms establishes equality before and under law and equal protection and benefit of law without discrimination based on, *inter alia*, age or mental or physical disability (Canadian Charter of Rights and Freedoms, 1982, Section 15).

The ideas that some citizens are better than others or that some ages in life are more beneficial to society are contrary to equal citizenship where all are equal. In practice, even legal protections can be insufficient to prevent the weakening of citizenship benefits with age. Laws, rules, social norms, policies and practices of societal institutions may unfairly restrict opportunities and create systemic or structural disadvantages for older people. For example, health-care rationing on the basis of age is widespread, and older adults tend to be excluded from medical research and data collection. Older workers are often disadvantaged in the workplace.

The disadvantaging of older individuals reduces their ability to participate fully in society by marginalizing them into a lower status. It also affects societies by eroding solidarity across ages and generations, which dilutes the fairness of the social contract between age groups. Negative or disqualifying attributes related to age can be used to define population categories. Acceptance of the disadvantaging of older individuals also suggests that the process of aging automatically leads to a status with unequal rights and fewer freedoms.

2.8.1 *Agism*

Agism is a negative force without a solid rationale, since normally everyone will live through all ages in the life course. With the increasing proportion of older people in national populations, reaching 25% and more, it is time to change the narrative around aging and human development. There are major economic and social costs to society if people in their later years are deprived of equal citizenship and the freedom to contribute to society.

Using age to stereotype individuals can lead to disadvantage, injustice and harm. Agism, particularly benevolent agism (patronizing), is often tolerated by society. Though both young and old can experience agism, it is not temporary for older people and the consequences can be long lasting and even cause loss of life. For older people, agism is associated with a shorter lifespan, poorer physical and mental health, slower recovery from disability and cognitive decline. Agism reduces the quality of life for people in later life. There are financial costs to societies, too. For example, the estimated cost of agism in the United States was US$ 63 billion per year in the period studied, or one of every seven dollars spent on eight health conditions for people 60 years and older (Levy et al., 2020).

2.9 Social Construction of the Phase of Later Life in Real Time

Longevity is a great achievement of our time, especially since it is a worldwide phenomenon. Legacy thinking of society still holds the traditional view of aging of the past century in its thrall despite the reality of this twenty-first century. Long lives are not the problem – rather it is living longer in societies designed for shorter lives.

Since transformation is in progress, social construction of lifelong human development has to be reimagined in real time. The social construction of aging entails the public understanding of the role and status of people in their later years as changes occur in society. The slow processes of social construction have to be speeded up to keep pace with societal changes to transform the role of people in later life and the way society works for all citizens.

The first insight is that later life is not a prolongation of middle age: the whole life course is a rearrangement of life events and experiences over a longer lifetime. Longevity is a gift of extra years, and time itself has to be managed as a resource rather than as background. Social roles can be changed and combined over longer lives. Understanding the impacts of longevity requires a life course perspective when determining intergenerational relationships and societal roles. People in later life have to be respected as survivors of multiple challenges over a long life, building knowledge and experience that will be transmitted to other generations. The disruption of past trends and traditional patterns are part of the dynamics of change that will shape future society.

The second insight is that the fluidity of culture in lived experience, rather than the rigidity of stereotypes from the past, must take precedence. Persons in their seventies and eighties today are very different from persons of that age 20 years ago. Society needs to understand what it means to live in a society with more old people than young in order to maximize the value arising from this new composition of its population. Culture should shape and form our society in ways that will embed valuable cultural elements at a time when more people are living longer and better lives. Citizens should look forward to aging into their later years. The population in their later lives will take their rightful place if society celebrates longevity.

References

AARP. (2022). *Global longevity economy outlook*. https://www.aarp.org/content/dam/aarp/research/surveys_statistics/econ/2022/global-longevity-economy-report.doi.10.26419-2Fint.00052.001.pdf

AARP Research. (2021). *2022 tech trends and the 50-plus* (Report). https://www.aarp.org/content/dam/aarp/research/surveys_statistics/technology/2021/2022-technology-trends-older-americans.doi.10.26419-2Fres.00493.001.pdf

AGE-WELL Network of Centres of Excellence (NCE). (2020, September 29). *Covid-19 has significantly increased the use of many technologies among older Canadians: Poll*. CISION. https://www.newswire.ca/news-releases/covid-19-has-significantly-increased-the-use-of-many-technologies-among-older-canadians-poll-865959030.html.

American Automobile Association. (n.d.). *Senior driver safety & mobility*. https://exchange.aaa.com/safety/senior-driver-safety-mobility/

Aung, M. N., Koyanagi, Y., Nagamine, Y., Nam, E. W., Mulati, N., Kyaw, M. Y., Moolphate, S., Shirayama, Y., Nonaka, K., Field, M., Cheung, P., & Yuasa, M. (2022). Digitally inclusive, healthy aging communities (DIHAC): A cross-cultural study in Japan, Republic of Korea, Singapore, and Thailand. *International Journal of Environmental Research and Public Health, 19*, Article 6976. https://doi.org/10.3390/ijerph19126976

Austin, P. L. (2019, July 25). What will smart homes look like 10 years from now? *Time*. https://time.com/5634791/smart-homes-future

BBC News. (2019, January 18). *Older drivers: Is age a factor behind the wheel?* https://www.bbc.com/news/uk-46916429

Bloom, D. E. (2020, March). *Population 2020*. International Monetary Fund, Finance and Development. https://www.elibrary.imf.org/view/journals/022/0057/001/022.0057.issue-001-en.xml

Bodner, E., Palgi, Y., & Wyman, M. F. (2018). Ageism in mental health assessment and treatment of older adults. In L. Ayalon & C. Tesch-Romer (Eds.), *Contemporary perspectives on ageism* (pp. 241–262). Springer. https://doi.org/10.1007/978-3-319-73820-8_15

Botes, R., Vermeulen, K. M., Correia, J., Buskens, E., & Janssen, F. (2018). Relative contribution of various chronic diseases and multi-morbidity to potential disability among Dutch elderly. *BMC Health Services Research, 18*(24), 1–8. https://doi.org/10.1186/s12913-017-2820-0

British Standards Institution. (2005, February 28). *New British standard addresses the need for inclusive design* [Press release]. https://www.bsigroup.com/en-GB/about-bsi/media-centre/press-releases/2005/2/New-British-Standard-addresses-the-need-for-inclusive-design/

Canadian Charter of Rights and Freedoms, Part I of the Constitution Act, 1982. *Justice Laws Website, Government of Canada*. https://laws-lois.justice.gc.ca/eng/Const/page-12.html

Caspi, A., Bern, D. J., & Elder, G. H. (1989). Continuities and consequences of interactional styles across the life course. *Journal of Personality, 57*(2), 375–406. https://doi.org/10.1111/j.1467-6494.1989.tb00487.x

Cheng, M. (2019, February 26). Grey divorce: Its reasons & its implications. *Forbes*. https://www.forbes.com/sites/margueritacheng/2019/02/26/grey-divorce-its-reasons-its-implications/?sh=179bc40d4acd

Christensen, K., Doblhammer, G., Rau, R., & Vaupel, J. W. (2009). Ageing populations: The challenges ahead. *Lancet, 374*(3696), 1196–1208. https://doi.org/10.1016/S0140-6736(09)61460-4

Deloitte. (2017). *2017 Global mobile consumer survey: US edition–The dawn of the next era in mobile*. https://www2.deloitte.com/content/dam/Deloitte/us/Documents/technology-media-telecommunications/us-tmt-2017-global-mobile-consumer-survey-executive-summary.pdf

Easterbrook, G. (2014, October). What happens when we all live to 100? *The Atlantic*. https://www.theatlantic.com/magazine/archive/2014/10/what-happens-when-we-all-live-to-100/379338/

Elder, G. H., Jr. (Ed.). (1985). *Life course dynamics: Trajectories and transitions, 1968–1980*. Cornell University Press.

Erikson, E. H. (1994). *Identity and the life cycle* [Reissued edition]. W.W. Norton.

Erikson, E. H., & Erikson, J. (1998). *The life cycle completed: Extended version with new chapters on the ninth stage of development*. W.W. Norton.

Eurostat. (2020). *Ageing Europe – Statistics on housing and living conditions*. Statistics Explained. https://ec.europa.eu/eurostat/statistics-explained/SEPDF/cache/80394.pdf

Faverio, M. (2022, January 13). Share of those 65 and older who are tech users has grown in the past decade. *Pew Research Center*. https://www.pewresearch.org/fact-tank/2022/01/13/share-of-those-65-and-older-who-are-tech-users-has-grown-in-the-past-decade/

GBD 2019 Dementia Forecasting Collaborators. (2022). Estimation of the global prevalence of dementia in 2019 and forecasted prevalence in 2050: an analysis for the Global Burden of Disease Study 2019. *The Lancet Public Health, 7*, e105–e125. https://doi.org/10.1016/S2468-2667(21)00249-8

George, S., & Choi, C. (2022, September 12). *Senior driving stats*. Finder. https://www.finder.com/elderly-driving-statistics

Government Office for Science. (2016). *Future of an ageing population*. United Kingdom. https://assets.publishing.service.gov.uk/government/uploads/system/uploads/attachment_data/file/816458/future-of-an-ageing-population.pdf

Gratton, L., & Scott, A. J. (2016). *The 100-year life: Living and working in an age of longevity*. Bloomsbury.

Gurrentz, B., & Mayol-Garcia, Y. (2021, April 22). *Marriage, divorce, widowhood remain prevalent among older populations*. United States Census Bureau. https://www.census.gov/library/stories/2021/04/love-and-loss-among-older-adults.html

Haight, B. K., Barba, B. E., Tesh, A. S., & Courts, N. F. (2002). Thriving: A life span theory. *Journal of Gerontological Nursing, 28*(3), 14–22. https://doi.org/10.3928/0098-9134-20020301-05

Hartshorne, J. K., & Germine, L. T. (2015). When does cognitive functioning peak? The asynchronous rise and fall of different cognitive abilities across the life span. *Psychological Science, 26*(4), 433–443. https://doi.org/10.1177/0956797614567339

Healthy Aging and Wellness Working Group. (2006). *Healthy aging in Canada: A new vision, a vital investment from evidence to action*. Background paper prepared for the federal, provincial and territorial Committee of Officials (Seniors). https://www.health.gov.bc.ca/library/publications/year/2006/Healthy_Aging_in_Canada_New_Vision_Vital_Investment_Discussion_Brief.pdf

Hersch, L. (1948). Démographie potentielle et vieillissement de la population [Potential demography and aging of the population]. *Population, 3*(2), 233–248. https://www.persee.fr/doc/pop_0032-4663_1948_num_3_2_1914

Hitlin, P. (2018, September 28). Internet, social media use and device ownership in U.S. have plateaued after years of growth. *Pew Research Center*. https://www.pewresearch.org/fact-tank/2018/09/28/internet-social-media-use-and-device-ownership-in-u-s-have-plateaued-after-years-of-growth/

Jeste, D. V., Depp, C. A., & Vahia, I. V. (2010). Successful cognitive and emotional aging. *World Psychiatry, 9*(2), 78–84. https://doi.org/10.1002/j.2051-5545.2010.tb00277.x

Klinenberg, E. (2012). *Going solo: The extraordinary rise and surprising appeal of living alone*. Penguin Books.

Kyriazis, M. (2016). *Challenging aging – The anti-senescence effects of hormesis, environmental enrichment and information exposure*. Bentham Books.

Lee, R., & Mason, A. (Eds.). (2011). *Population aging and the generational economy: A global perspective*. Edward Elgar and International Development Research Centre.

Leon, M., & Woo, C. (2018). Environmental enrichment and successful aging. *Frontiers in Behavioral Neuroscience, 12*, Article 155. https://doi.org/10.3389/fnbeh.2018.00155

Levy, B. R., Slade, M. D., Chang, E.-S., Kannoth, S., & Wang, S.-Y. (2020). Ageism amplifies cost and prevalence of health conditions. *The Gerontologist, 60*(1), 174–181. https://doi.org/10.1093/geront/gny131

Lim, J. K. H., Li, Q.-X., He, Z., Vingrys, A. J., Wong, V. H. Y., Currier, N., Mullen, J., Bui, B. V., & Nguyen, C. T. O. (2016). The eye as a biomarker for Alzheimer's disease. *Frontiers in Neuroscience, 10*, Article 536. https://doi.org/10.3389/fnins.2016.00536

Livingston, G. (2019, June 18). Americans 60 and older are spending more time in front of their screens than a decade ago. *Pew Research Center*. https://www.pewresearch.org/fact-tank/2019/06/18/americans-60-and-older-are-spending-more-time-in-front-of-their-screens-than-a-decade-ago/

Maier, H., Gampe, J., Jeune, B., Robine, J.-M., & Vaupel, J. W. (Eds.). (2010). *Supercentenarians*. Springer.

Molteni, R., Zheng, J.-Q., Ying, Z., Gómez-Pinilla, F., & Twiss, J. L. (2004). Voluntary exercise increases axonal regeneration from sensory neurons. *Proceedings of the National Academy of Sciences, USA, 101*(22), 8473–8478. https://doi.org/10.1073/pnas.040144310

Moody, H. R. (2008). Eco-elders: Legacy and environmental advocacy. *Generations, 33*(4), 70–74. https://www.jstor.org/stable/26555704

Morris, S., Fawcett, G., Brisebois, L., & Hughes, J. (2018) *A demographic, employment and income profile of Canadians with disabilities aged 15 years and over, 2017*. Statistics Canada, Canadian Survey on Disability. https://www150.statcan.gc.ca/n1/pub/89-654-x/89-654-x2018002-eng.htm

No Isolation. (2018, June 22). *Why do many seniors have trouble using technology?* https://www.noisolation.com/global/research/why-do-many-seniors-have-trouble-using-technology/

OECD. (2019a). *Society at a glance 2019: OECD social indicators*. OECD Publishing. https://doi.org/10.1787/soc_glance-2019-en

OECD. (2019b). *Working better with age: Ageing and employment policies*. OECD Publishing. https://doi.org/10.1787/c4d4f66a-en

Office of Highway Policy Information. (2018). *Highway statistics 2018*. Federal Highway Administration (USA). https://www.fhwa.dot.gov/policyinformation/statistics/2021/

Ogg, J., & Renaut, S. (2006). The support of parents in old age by those born during 1945–1954: A European perspective. *Ageing & Society, 26*(5), 723–743. https://doi.org/10.1017/S0144686X06004922

Oldest Living People. (2023, March 13). In *Gerontology Wiki*. https://gerontology.fandom.com/wiki/Oldest_living_people

Population Division. (2002). *World population ageing: 1950–2050*. ST/ESA/SER.A/207. United Nations. https://digitallibrary.un.org/record/461899?ln=en

Population Division. (2019). *World population ageing 2019: Highlights* (ST/ESA/SER.A/430). United Nations. https://www.un.org/en/development/desa/population/publications/pdf/ageing/WorldPopulationAgeing2019-Highlights.pdf

Population Division. (2022). *Life expectancy at birth* [Data portal]. United Nations. Retrieved 6 January 2023. https://population.un.org/dataportal/data/indicators/61/locations/900/start/1960/end/2022/table/pivotbylocation

President's Council of Advisors on Science and Technology. (2016). *Independence, technology, and connection in older age*. https://obamawhitehouse.archives.gov/sites/default/files/microsites/ostp/PCAST/pcast_independence_tech__aging_report_final_0.pdf

Public Health Agency of Canada. (2020). *Aging and chronic diseases: A profile of Canadian seniors*. https://www.canada.ca/en/public-health/services/publications/diseases-conditions/aging-chronic-diseases-profile-canadian-seniors-executive-summary.html

Reher, D., & Requena, M. (2018). Living alone in later life: A global perspective. *Population and Development Review, 44*(3), 427–454. https://doi.org/10.1111/padr.12149

Reini, K., & Saarela, J. (2021). Life expectancy of the ethnically mixed: Register-based evidence from native Finns. *International Journal of Environmental Research and Public Health, 18*(7), Article 3415. https://doi.org/10.3390/ijerph18073415

Roberts, Y. (2014, June 15). It's never too late to say 'I do': why the over-65s have fallen for marriage. *The Guardian.* https://www.theguardian.com/society/2014/jun/15/why-over-65s-have-fallen-for-marriage

Sanderson, W. C., & Scherbov, S. (2019). *Prospective longevity: A new vision of population aging.* Harvard University Press.

Schwarzinger, M., & Dufouil, C. (2022). Forecasting the prevalence of dementia. *The Lancet Public Health, 7*(2), e94–e95. https://doi.org/10.1016/S2468-2667(21)00277-2

Seabrook, A. (2008, June 7). *Tip-of-tongue moments reveal brain's organization* [Interview]. NPR Science Out of the Box. https://www.npr.org/templates/story/story.php?storyId=91284151

Shephard, R. J. (1998). Aging and exercise. In T. D. Fahey (Ed.), *Encyclopedia of sports medicine and science.* Internet Society for Sport Science. https://www.sportsci.org/encyc/agingex/agingex.html

SilverEco. (2018, July 12). *In 2030, ¼ of European drivers will be over 65 years old.* http://www.silvereco.org/en/in-2030-1-4-of-european-drivers-will-be-over-65-years-old/

Sinha, S. K. (2020, October 13). *Almost 100 per cent of older Canadians surveyed plan to live independently in their own homes, but is this even possible?* National Institute on Ageing. https://www.nia-ryerson.ca/commentary-posts/2020/9/22/almost-100-per-cent-of-older-canadians-surveyed-plan-to-live-independently-in-their-own-homes-but-is-this-even-possible

Slettemeås, D., Mainsah, H., & Berg, L. (2018). *Eldres digitale hverdag. En landsdekkende undersøkelse om tilgang, mestring og utfordringer i informasjonssamfunnet* [Elderly's digital daily life. A nationwide study of access, management and challenges in the information society]. Oslo Met og SIFO oppdragsrapport nr. 18-2018. https://oda.oslomet.no/oda-xmlui/handle/20.500.12199/1309

Smith, A. (2014, April 3). Attitudes, impacts and barriers to adoption. *Pew Research Center.* https://www.pewresearch.org/internet/2014/04/03/attitudes-impacts-and-barriers-to-adoption/

Statistics Canada. (2022a). *A portrait of Canada's growing population aged 85 and older from the 2021 census.* Census in Brief. https://www12.statcan.gc.ca/census-recensement/2021/as-sa/98-200-X/2021004/98-200-X2021004-eng.pdf

Statistics Canada. (2022b, August 22). *Projected population, by projection scenario, age and sex, as of July 1* [Data portal]. https://www150.statcan.gc.ca/t1/tbl1/en/tv.action?pid=1710005701&pickMembers%5B0%5D=1.1&pickMembers%5B1%5D=3.1&pickMembers%5B2%5D=4.202&cubeTimeFrame.startYear=2021&cubeTimeFrame.endYear=2050&referencePeriods=20210101%2C20500101

Statistics Canada. (2022c). *Smokers, by age group* (Table 13-10-0096-10). https://www150.statcan.gc.ca/t1/tbl1/en/tv.action?pid=1310009610

Statistisches Bundesamt. (2022, December 2). *4 million more people aged 67 or over will live in Germany in 2035* (Press release No. 511). Destatis. https://www.destatis.de/EN/Press/2022/12/PE22_511_124.html

Steele, A. (2020). *Ageless: The new science of getting older without getting old.* Bloomsbury.

Stepler, R. (2016, April 21). World's centenarian population projected to grow eightfold by 2050. *Pew Research Center.* https://www.pewresearch.org/fact-tank/2016/04/21/worlds-centenarian-population-projected-to-grow-eightfold-by-2050/

Sundström, G., Johansson, L., & Hassing, L. B. (2002). The shifting balance of long-term care in Sweden. *The Gerontologist, 42*(3), 350–355. https://doi.org/10.1093/geront/42.3.350

Tang, J., Galbraith, N., & Truong, J. (2019). *Living alone in Canada.* Statistics Canada, Insights on Canadian Society. https://www150.statcan.gc.ca/n1/pub/75-006-x/2019001/article/00003-eng.htm

Tornstam, L. (1994). Gerotranscendence: A theoretical and empirical exploration. In L. E. Thomas & S. A. Eisenhandler (Eds.), *Aging and the religious dimension* (pp. 203–225). Greenwood.

Turcotte, M. (2012). *Profile of seniors' transportation habits*. Statistics Canada, Canadian Social Trends. https://www150.statcan.gc.ca/n1/pub/11-008-x/2012001/article/11619-eng.htm

United Health Foundation. (2022). *America's health rankings. 2022 Senior Report.* https://www.americashealthrankings.org/learn/reports/2022-senior-report

United Nations. (1948). *Universal declaration of Human Rights*. https://www.un.org/en/about-us/universal-declaration-of-human-rights

United States Census Bureau. (2011, May 18). *Census Bureau reports 55 percent have married one time* (News release). https://www.census.gov/newsroom/releases/archives/marital_status_living_arrangements/cb11-90.html

United States Census Bureau. (2019, March 13). *Older people projected to outnumber children for the first time in U.S. history* (Press release Number CB18-41. Revised 2019, October 8). https://www.census.gov/newsroom/press-releases/2018/cb18-41-population-projections.html

WARC. (2020, January 29). *Samsung looks to 'inclusive design' to reach boomers*. https://www.warc.com/newsandopinion/news/samsung-looks-to-inclusive-design-to-reach-boomers/43166

Watson, K. B., Carlson, S. A., Gunn, J. P., Galuska, D. A., O'Connor, A., Greenlund, K. J., & Fulton, J. E. (2016). Physical inactivity among adults aged 50 years and older – United States, 2014. *Morbidity and Mortality Weekly Report, 65*(36), 954–958. https://doi.org/10.15585/mmwr.mm6536a3

White Riley, M., Johnson, M., & Foner, A. (1972). *A sociology of age stratification. Volume 3 of aging and society*. Russel Sage. https://www.russellsage.org/sites/default/files/AgingSociety-vol3download.pdf

White Riley, M., Khan, R. L., & Foner, A. (Eds.). (1994). *Age and structural lag: Failure to provide opportunities in work, family and leisure*. Wiley.

Widmer, E. D., & Ritschard, G. (2009). The de-standardization of the life course: Are men and women equal? *Advances in Life Course Research, 14*(1–2), 28–39. https://www.sciencedirect.com/science/article/abs/pii/S1040260809000069

Wolters, F. J., Chibnik, L. B., Waziry, R., Anderson, R., Berr, C., Beiser, A., Bis, J. C., Blacker, D., Bos, D., Brayne, C., Dartigues, J.-F., Darweesh, S. K. L., Davis-Plourde, K. L., de Wolf, F., Debette, S., Dufouil, C., Fornage, M., Goudsmit, J., Grasset, L., et al. (2020). Twenty-seven-year time trends in dementia incidence in Europe and the United States. *Neurology, 95*(5), e519–e531. https://n.neurology.org/content/95/5/e519

World Health Organization. (2022, September 20). *Dementia. Fact sheets*. https://www.who.int/news-room/fact-sheets/detail/dementia

Chapter 3
Societal Gains from a Larger Population Share of Older People

3.1 Can Society Benefit from Greater Longevity?

Unequivocally, the response is yes, it can. The question is not whether but how much? If increased longevity results in lives of purpose, where older persons continue to contribute to society in ways that are simply related to two more decades of later life, society will benefit. But the greater gain is from the longevity dividend. In a society that makes the right decisions, the gains from greater longevity are both short and long term – for current living generations and future generations.

Demographic preparedness is key. Awareness of population aging is not by itself enough, since it can lead to complacency and reliance on past attitudes and policies. Individuals and society must make the effort to understand the opportunities that increased longevity presents and engage in coordinated action to benefit from them.

Greater longevity has resulted in decades of life after work for a large proportion of the population. Longer lifetimes have caused a break in traditional patterns and pathways of the life course, resulting in societal transformation. This new phase of life merits a fair and just role in society and a status commensurate to its place in the life course. A proper life course perspective would consider societal responsibilities for this life stage based on capabilities gained over the lifetime.

The social compact has to be re-designed to be made meaningful in the new context. The lifetime balance of investments and costs relative to societal contributions should be examined. Later life has an undeserved reputation because its value is burdened by past ideas of dependency ratios and the tendency to measure contributions by outdated criteria that apply primarily to the working years. Furthermore, there is a tendency both to use only economic and labour market factors rather than broader ones and to apply them to the later years rather than to the entire life course.

Social policies that were designed when there were fewer older people are now less effective. Policies and societal institutions underperform because they were designed for a differently composed population and for a different economic and

S. Brink, *The Longevity Dividend*, International Perspectives on Aging 39,
https://doi.org/10.1007/978-3-031-35335-2_3

social pattern of exchange over the life course. The lack of a life course perspective in policy development resulted in short-term goals and long-term unintended consequences. For instance, instead of investing more in primary and preventive care, which would keep people healthy through life, health expenditures are heavily skewed to acute and hospital care, which is often too little too late. Rather than favouring aging in place with home care, which is better and cheaper for most older persons, the only option available to those who need care and support may be expensive long term care residences.

The life course perspective recognizes that people's contributions can vary in content and intensity over the life span, with peaks and ebbs, rather than progressively declining with age after early adulthood. A realistic understanding of the contributions of people in later life indicates that they are underestimated while their consumption of public services is overestimated. As noted earlier, contributive justice matches a person's obligations with his or her capabilities and role in society (Sandel, 2020) without diminishing the responsibility of citizens to contribute to collective wellbeing and progress appropriate to their age and circumstance.

3.2 Negative Perceptions of Aging Lead People in Later Life to Underestimate Their Own Contributions

Though most people in the later years of life are healthy, active and contributing members of society, they are widely considered to be fragile and incompetent to manage modern life. The public perception of aging and older people tends towards negative rather than positive images, contrary to reality. An older person may use a wheel chair but can still participate in the economy and society.

People in later life are altered by aging, but they should not be compared to younger generations or even to their younger selves. Despite the great diversity among older people, stereotypes prevail. It is common to describe older people by using negative attributes such as cranky, forgetful or senile. People in later life are judged by the weakest among them, and entire cohorts are considered to be less valuable to society.

Negative characteristics applied to a whole group can affect the life chances of individuals. Older people are considered to resist change or be slow to learn and adapt to modern life and, consequently, considered not to be productive or active. This perception can lead older people themselves to feel less valuable to society. A study of older adults found that about a third of older survey respondents thought they were incompetent and had nothing to contribute (Table 3.1). This is a most pernicious impact of agism against a whole segment of the population.

Table 3.1 Perception of people in later life experiencing agism with negative consequences

Statements	Agreeing with statement
People have assumed I have nothing to contribute	38%
People have assumed I'm incompetent	27%

Reproduced from Revera report on ageism by Revera and International Federation of Aging (2012) with permission from International Federation of Aging.

In contrast, positive attitudes towards people in later life and a culture that values aging as part of human development will imbue older people with a sense of purpose and society with optimism. Levy et al. (2002) found that older people with more positive self-perceptions of aging tended to live 7.5 years longer than those with less positive perceptions. The contribution made by people during their later lives should be recognized and not underestimated. Such contributions made by the much larger numbers of older people results eventually in the longevity dividend as described in later chapters.

3.3 Productive Contributions by People in Their Later Years

Productive contributions, whether tangible or intangible, are those that increase growth, reduce costs or foster social progress of society. Contrary to public perception, many older people perform multiple roles simultaneously in their lives – worker, mentor, grandparent, consumer, investor and volunteer (Guberman et al., 2012). When older adults are able and have the opportunity, they contribute to every societal institution – economy, social relations, civil society and government – in ways that improve the quality of life of contemporary and future generations (Mei et al., 2013). It is relevant to note that the exchange of services and contributions to society is a two-way exchange.

3.3.1 Longevity Economy

Secure economic status is related to positive health and social outcomes for people in later life. This determines their activity by affecting their consumption patterns, leisure activities and investments. The Longevity Economy, also called the Silver Economy, represents the sum of all economic activity that serves the needs of people over 50. It includes both the products and services that they purchase directly and the further economic activity that this spending generates in addition to their contributions of economic value. Though the consumption patterns may differ, people in later life contribute to the Silver Economy.

The Longevity Economy is an often underappreciated part of the economy. Relative to their percentage of the total population, older people generate a disproportionately large share of Gross Domestic Product (GDP) through their spending on goods and services. In 2020 the global population aged over 50 years contributed as much as 34% of global GDP while accounting for only about 24% of the world population (AARP, 2022). The share of GDP is expected to continue to grow. The contribution to the global GDP made by the 50-plus population could rise to US$ 65 trillion or 36% by 2030, possibly continuing to rise to 39% by 2050.

The Longevity Economy is a predictable growing international phenomenon. The Silver Economy project of the European Union estimated that Europeans over 65 had a spending capacity of over € 3 trillion (European Commission, 2017). While the total yearly spending power of older consumers is quite equally distributed across Asia, North America, and Europe, it is likely to shift from the OECD economies to emerging markets, especially to Asia (Fengler, 2021). The difference in estimated future yearly growth rates of 0.8% for the world population for some years and 3.2% for older persons will increase the relative size of the Silver Economy. The potential economic role of the population 50 years and over could be significant also in low or middle income countries. Estimates range from 26% of GDP in Ethiopia to 56% in Cambodia by 2050 (AARP, 2022).

Consumption

In terms of the share of GDP represented by consumption, in 2020 people in the 50-plus group accounted for half of global consumption spending (AARP, 2022). This share could grow to 59% by 2050 (US$ 96 trillion). In Japan, for example, where consumer spending is the biggest component of the national economy, people over the age of 65 contribute almost 40% of consumer spending, in contrast to making up 29% of the population (Fujioka, 2020).

The major areas of consumption spending include health, housing and leisure and hospitality. The increasing consumption spending by the 50-plus group benefits their families and communities where they live.

Savings and Investment

The current older generation has the reputation of being the wealthiest in history. The post-war baby boomer generation was financially prudent. In Canada, the wealth of older people quadrupled since 1984, which outpaced the growth of wealth among younger generations (McMahon, 2018). In the United States, the Federal Reserve's Survey of Consumer Finances captured the shift of wealth to those 75 and over in comparison to younger families between 2013 and 2016 (Howe, 2018). Where once the rates of poverty were high, today's older persons are well off compared to previous older generations. Financial discipline, aggressive saving, and risk averse investing, particularly in housing, among older people combined with stock market booms, reliable economic growth, soaring real estate values and better pension coverage contribute to this development.

However, the distribution of wealth is uneven and not all people over 75 are prosperous, or even homeowners. Persons over 75 live for the most part on fixed incomes, and though they may have savings, they may lack liquidity. For those who own their primary residence, this is often their main savings instrument. If they do not wish to sell, many older people thus find themselves house rich but income poor. Instruments to use the home to create an income stream exist, but many older people are leery of using them.

The savings of older people may yield poor returns, requiring them to draw down their savings. Many older people rely on income from investments to supplement their basic public pensions. Funds held in savings accounts have sometimes generated only low interest income or none at all. Older people often are or are thought to be less well informed about money management, including such features as internet banking or crypto investments. This can make them vulnerable to credit card fraud and other scams.

3.3.2 Paid Work

Retirement options in many cases now include flexibility that encourages bridging through different forms of work and part-time employment. This allows older people to ease into retirement while employers can benefit from their experience and knowledge for longer. People are working more years and in later life may work at a different pace and rhythm. Others are starting a new career as entrepreneurs, artists, writers and consultants.

The share of older workers among those employed can be significant. In Canada, one in five people 65 or over worked at some point during the year 2016 (Statistics Canada, 2017). Thirty percent of these nearly 1.1 million older people worked the full year and full-time and the rest for part year or part-time. Two major groups of older people were more likely to work: those with a bachelor's degree or higher and those without private retirement income. In Sweden, the employment rate for those 60–64 was 75% in 2015, one of the highest rates in Europe (Laun & Palme, 2017). Though the rate falls with higher age, the rate was still 26% for those 65–69.

Globally, 3.7% of the labour force were workers 65 years and over in 2015 and the proportion is expected to rise to 5.3% in 2030 (Department of Statistics, 2018). This is a faster increase than in the past few decades. The share of youth (aged 15–24) is expected to continue its steady decrease. The accelerating change in the age distribution of the labour force underscores the importance of integrating older workers better by matching their expectations with labour market needs and by reorganizing work and retirement arrangements.

The global trends are evident also in national labour force projections. In the United States, it is projected that 8.2% of workers in the labour force will be aged over 65 in 2024, compared to only 3.4% in 2004. Their labour participation rate is expected to increase the fastest for people aged 65–75 and 75 and older (Toossi & Torpey, 2017). Older American workers play a major role in the job market and the economy. In 2018, 88.6 million jobs (44% of total employment) were held or created by people 50 and over, and the economic contributions of this group totaled US$ 8.3 trillion (Terrell, 2019).

However, around the world, many older people are unable to retire. Nearly half of all people over pensionable age do not receive a pension or receive pensions that are inadequate (Social Protection Department, 2014). They subsist by continuing to work, often in low wage precarious jobs, to supplement their public income assistance.

Self-Employment and Entrepreneurship

Older people are a significant entrepreneurial resource with competencies that are often overlooked and undervalued (Fig. 3.1). Besides offering unemployed older people an opportunity to work on something of interest, third-age entrepreneurship has the potential to enhance the innovative capacity of the economy by employing the human and social capital of mature individuals through new pioneering start-ups. Older people also have some inherent advantages compared to younger entrepreneurs, such as more developed networks, more work and industry experience, higher technical and managerial skill levels, and a stronger financial position (Botham & Graves, 2009).

Older people are considered to be technologically uninformed. However, there is evidence that entrepreneurs 65 and over were just as likely to use online crowd funding as younger entrepreneurs (Schøtt et al., 2017). They also used their personal savings to finance their business.

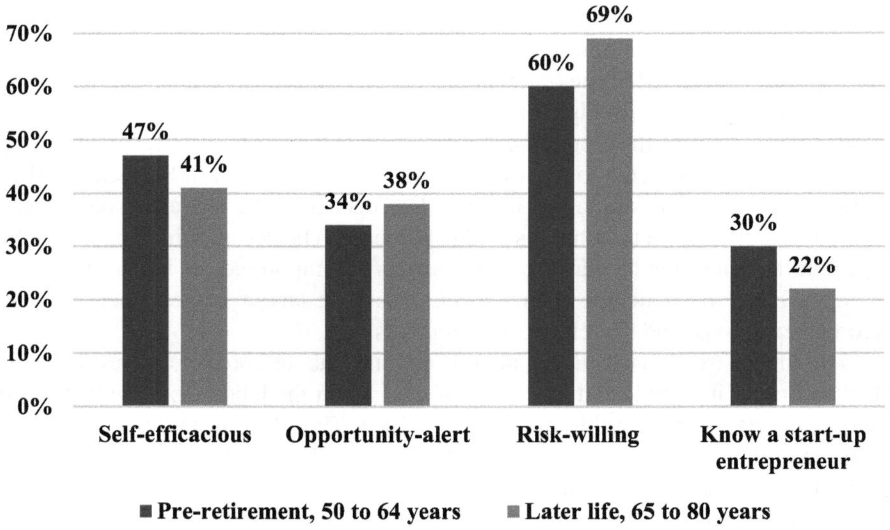

Fig. 3.1 Advantageous entrepreneurial competencies of older adults by age, 2017
(Data from Senior Entrepreneurship – Special topic report 2016–2017 by Schøtt et al. (2017, Figure 2.2). Reproduced with permission from Global Entrepreneurship Monitor)

Though entrepreneurial support and programs are often geared towards younger people, the highest rate of business start-up activity in the United States is among those aged 55–64. People aged 60-plus now comprise over one third of new entrepreneurs in Japan. In the United Kingdom, 'third age' entrepreneurs are responsible for over a quarter of new start-ups. (Davey, 2021). Similar trends are noted in Australia and New Zealand.

Many older people choose self-employment as a late-career option because it is a flexible alternative to organizational employment, offers opportunities for self-managed work-life balance, generates additional income for retirement and later years or allows the individual to maintain their preferred lifestyle despite prejudices against older entrepreneurs (Kibler et al., 2015). Globally, 13% of adults between the ages of 65 and 80 are self-employed, compared to just 11% of adults 18–29 years old (Schøtt et al., 2017).

3.3.3 Exchanges and Transfers

Exchanges and transfers can be financial or social and generally occur within the family and between generations but sometimes between friends. They can be activities that have economic value and can be tangible or intangible. They are motivated by relationships and values rather than by contract.

Inheritances

People in the well-to-do generation in later life are getting older, retiring and dying. The millennial generation in the United States was estimated in 2019 to inherit roughly US$ 68 trillion from their baby boomer parents by 2030 (Kelly, 2019). This intergenerational transfer will be a boon to the younger generation, which did not have the advantageous conditions for earning, saving or investing of the previous generation. The transfer is exceptional because of the favourable economic circumstances parents experienced in their adult years. Such large transfers are not expected to always continue from parents to children in the future.

Parents' Economic and Other Support of Adult Children

Parents often provide economic support to adult children as they undertake higher education, enter the labour market and start a household. Support can range from sharing costs, such as living with parents and subsidizing costs including education fees or housing mortgages (Cobb-Clark & Gørgens, 2014). It could also include assistance such as using parent's social networks, transfer of a family car and mentoring.

3.3.4 *Care Economy*

The care economy makes an important contribution to the smooth functioning of societies by linking those that need care and nurturing and those that provide it, whether paid or unpaid.

Self-Care

Self-care is important for healthy and active aging. Digitally savvy older people get health advice from the internet for diet, exercise and minor discomforts and ailments. Maintaining their health saves money for both individuals and public health agencies. Well informed self-care reduces demand for home care services and saves substantial out of pocket spending. In the United States, among those 65 and older, 74% could fund at least 2 years of paid moderate home care if they liquidated all their assets (Johnson & Wang, 2019). The oldest and sickest are, regrettably, most likely to have insufficient income to afford paid home care.

Interestingly, even older people who do not make other contributions provide a societal benefit by achieving better health through self-care not paid for by others. In Europe, self-care is estimated to save health systems and national economies € 34 billion a year, though there are variations in levels of self-care among countries (May & Bauer, 2021).

Grandparenting and Family or Kinship Care

The role of grandparenting has grown with the longevity trend. Estimates by the Max Planck Institute using UN data found that there were 1.5 billion grandparents in the world ("The age of the grandparent has arrived", 2023). The ratio of grandparents to children under 15 has grown from 0.46 in 1960 to 0.8 in 2023. Older people are healthier and, since they have fewer grandchildren, they can have a closer relationship with them. Grandparents and even great grandparents are able to have longer and closer relationships with their young descendants. In Canada, in 2011, the average estimated duration of grandparenthood was 24.3 years for grandmothers, who typically live longer, and 18.9 years for grandfathers (Margolis, 2016). Some live long enough to attend the weddings of their grandchildren and to hold their great grandchildren. Many have a close relationship with grandchildren, helping with child rearing, driving, and school work to support the working parents. Since women live longer, their roles range from 'granny as nanny' to sole caretaker of a grandchild. Grandmothers play an important role in caring for children, particularly in immigrant and ethnic families (Statistics Canada, 2019).

The share of grandparents aged 85 and over is increasing in Canada. This share almost tripled between 1995 and 2017, rising from 3 to 8% of grandparents (Statistics Canada, 2019). Grandmothers outnumbered grandfathers in 2019, with

4.2 million grandmothers, compared to 3.3 million grandfathers. In 2016, there were about 404,000 multi-generational or three-plus generations living together in Canada. This fast-growing household type accounted for 5% of households. About 32,520 children under the age of 14 lived under the sole care of their grandparents (without parents), in a 'skip-generation household' (Vanier Institute of the Family, 2019).

Skip-generation households increased also in low and middle income countries from 1.7% to 2.4% of households between 1990 and 2016 (Zimmer & Treleaven, 2020). In South Africa, grandparents assume the care of grandchildren orphaned by the death of parents due to HIV (Mtshali, 2016). Skip-generation households save the public costs of caring for orphans and, moreover, well raised children are thought to contribute more to society as adults.

Care of children by relatives or even close family friends is referred to as kinship care. They are often empty nest older family members who accept this responsibility. Kinship care provides stable child rearing in a permanent home, resulting in better outcomes for children, and in the long term benefits society and the economy. Such care, instead of foster care, saves the public purse in England an estimated £ 40,000 per child per year (Nicol Economics, 2020). Long term benefits result in healthier and better educated children, who engage less in anti-social behaviour or crime.

Caregiving

The need for caregiving services for people in later life is escalating at a fast rate because of the rapid growth of the older population. There will be more older people in need of care without children to care for them, but also fewer people of caregiving age to work as informal or professional caregivers for older people, whether in collective dwellings or at home. In OECD countries, there were about 4 people of working age (15–64 years) on average for each person 65 years and over in 2012, but it is projected to fall to 2 people in the next 40 years (OECD, 2020). By 2050, the proportion of people aged 80 and over (when they are likely to receive at least some care from others) in OECD countries will increase from nearly 5% to around 10% of the population on average. In Canada, the estimated number of older people requiring care services is expected to double over the next 20 years (Living Assistance Services, 2019).

Naturally occurring care relationships can also form between unpaid, non-professional caregivers and frail older people living in the community. In the United States, of all carers providing care, 10% cared for a friend, neighbour or non-relative (AARP & National Alliance for Caregiving, 2020). This is indicative of the number of fragile older people who need care but do not have access to family carers. A gap is being filled by an insecure but valuable source of care that is often unrecognized.

The economic value of unpaid caregivers is large. The annual economic value of the unpaid care provided in Canada by 7.8 million caregivers was estimated to be C$ 97 billion in 2018. This represented 4.2% of GDP and one third of national expenditures on health care (Research on aging – Policies and Practice, 2022). In the United States, informal home care had an estimated economic value of US$ 470 billion in 2013, which exceeded the costs of paid home care and Medicare (Living Assistance Services, 2019).

Many of the caregivers are aged over 65 themselves and they are getting older. One quarter of Canadian adults 65 years and over were caregivers (Arriagada, 2020). In Canada, of the 7.8 million caregivers, many are spouses caring for their partners and others are adult children in their sixties (one million are over 65 years old) and seventies, caring for parents aged 85 and over (Statistics Canada, 2020a). In the United States, 7% of caregivers are 75 years and over (AARP & National Alliance for Caregiving, 2020). Of these caregivers aged 75 and over, 74% provide care for a recipient of a similar age. Most of them are women. The average duration of the caregiving role is 4.5 years.

The simplistic reaction to the growing demand for care has been to promote increases in home care and formal caregiving. Besides difficulties stemming from labour scarcity, the results are likely to be sub-optimal. Ideally, if sufficient people are available, the care and support that older people need should be reallocated between those who are best able to provide each different type of care, instead of all care being delivered by a person from one source. Families are best able to provide love and affective care and maintain links to social networks. Professionals should provide the care which enables health and independence. A third group would supply home cleaning, snow clearing, maintenance and repairs. This would have the added advantage of splitting the effort and costs between family, private and public sectors.

3.3.5 Civil Society

Civil society (the non-profit sector) comprises individuals, groups or organizations that are not private sector business or government and who work for the betterment and advancement of members, the disadvantaged or society as a whole. Older people have been known to contribute informally to the unrecorded 'grey economy'.

Volunteering

In many countries, older people contribute considerable hours of unpaid volunteer work. In Australia, 2.2 million older people donated an average of around 411.9 hours a year (Della Bosca, 2018).

In Canada, older people volunteered more time per person than any other age group in 2018 (Hahmann et al., 2020). Though more of those 55–75 years were involved in formal volunteering (39%) a surprisingly large number of those 75 and over were involved, too (32%). This latter group volunteered on average over

200 hours per year. The numbers involved in informal volunteering were even higher: 73% of persons 55–75 and 58% of those 75 and over.

Charities and non-profit organizations play a vital role in supporting and enriching the lives of people in their communities. Most of them have volunteer boards and, in Canada, 22% of board members were aged 65 or older (Statistics Canada, 2021).

The monetary value of the volunteer work by older people is considerable. In the United States, people 50 years and over contributed US$ 745 billion worth of unpaid activities in 2018 in ways that help society in general (Terrell, 2019). The volunteer efforts of Canadian older people have generated more than C$ 10.9 billion in economic value (Revera, 2019). In 2018, the news warned that Australia would face an economic disaster if older people stopped volunteering, since their efforts were valued at as much as A$ 46.5 billion (Della Bosca, 2018).

Charitable Contributions

Not every person over 75 can volunteer. However, 90% of Canadians 65 and older believe they play a significant role in contributing to solving major world issues (Revera, 2019). Many persons in later life both donate money and volunteer their time. About 82% said they donate, and more than one-third (37%) volunteer time. Canadian tax filers 65 years and older donated C$ 4.8 billion in 2020, accounting for 45% of the total donated amount (Statistics Canada, 2022c). The average amount of their donations was C$ 2890, which exceeds the national average by 40%. These donors, 65 years and older, constituted 32% of all tax filer donors, a percentage that has increased since 2010. Charitable contributions are made regardless of age and living arrangements. It is likely that those who cannot volunteer continue to make charitable donations.

Social Entrepreneurship and Informal Investment

Older individuals often start, lead or participate in activities, organizations or initiatives that have social, community or environmental objectives and which exhibit social entrepreneurship. This could include a variety of self-help (training), community action (visiting at risk older people) or environmental activities (reducing waste). There is evidence that 8% of older adults are social entrepreneurs (Schøtt et al., 2017).

Older people also are likely to make informal investments and to serve as generous 'business angels'. They tend to invest more money compared to younger adults (Schøtt et al., 2017). Almost two thirds of older business angels invest more than the median of all investments. They often invest in a new business of a family member, but they also fund a stranger who has a good business idea.

3.3.6 *Political Institutions and Government*

Tax Contributions

Older people with low incomes benefit from income support programs and tax relief in many countries. Most older people also contribute to government revenue, even if only through consumption taxes, such as sales taxes or value added taxes. They may pay residential or municipal taxes and, if they have higher incomes, also income tax.

Though there is little data on the tax contributions of individuals in the later life stage, there is evidence that, in most countries, the young and the old pay less taxes than the middle age groups. However, their contribution is sizeable. In Canada individuals aged 35–54 years were 37% of tax filers and paid 52.4% of all income taxes in 2008 (Froats, 2011). Individuals aged 65 years and over constituted 18% of tax filers and paid 12.5% of income taxes. Those under 25 composed about 13% of tax filers but only contributed 2.2% of income taxes. In the United States, tax filers in the 35–54 years age group were 39% of tax filers with a tax liability in 2008 and paid 50% of total income taxes (Statistics of Income Division, 2023, Table 3.7). Tax filers 65 years and over accounted for 15% of tax returns and paid 16% of all income taxes. About two-thirds of this age group paid income tax. Those under 26 years paid 2% of total income taxes. In Germany, in 2016, the 'tax burden' for those between 18–24 years was 7.3%, while it was 7.0% for those 65 years and over (Beznoska & Hentze, 2017).

Savings to Public Budgets Without Compromising Quality of Life in Later Life

Some living arrangements in later life offer good examples of potential savings to public budgets. Savings can accrue from delayed aging through better health and aging in place as long as possible with the help of family care and even publicly funded home care. Reliance on nursing home care at later ages for only those who need it and for shorter time periods also saves public funds.

Healthy aging saves financial costs for both individuals and society. In the United States, one 'delayed aging' scenario would see social benefits amounting to US$ 7 trillion over 50 years (Goldman et al., 2013). Public policy goals and the desires of older people to age in place coincide. Almost 100% of Canadians 65 and over plan to age in their own homes, supporting themselves to live safely and independently as long as possible (Sinha & Nolan, 2020).

Older people who are helped to age in place through well formulated proactive policies may enable major savings to tax payers. A higher proportion of people aging in place yields savings for more individuals and gives them autonomy and life satisfaction. If older people are healthier due to supportive policies, the number of older people living at home can rise. About 75% of Danes 65 and over age at home with the help of home care services (OECD, 2021). In other countries, there are long waiting lists in collective settings because of inadequate home care. Saving on homecare and paying for nursing home care may be false economy. The cost to build and operate nursing homes and care homes will be exorbitant because of the growth of the older population. To develop a long-term care bed costs between C$ 212,000 and C$ 268,000 in Ontario, Canada (Sinha & Nolan, 2020). Providing care to a person aging in place costs about C$ 103 per day in Canada, whereas care for a nursing home resident costs about C$ 200 per day. Roughly 10–20% of older people would benefit from home care. At 0.2% of GDP, spending on home care in Canada is the second lowest among OECD countries (Drummond et al., 2020).

Delaying nursing home care as long as possible, while maintaining quality of life, saves public and private costs. Among centenarians in Canada, 54% lived in collective dwellings, such as nursing homes and care homes, and 85% of these centenarians were women (Statistics Canada, 2022a). The remaining older people lived autonomously. In the United States, 36% of nursing home residents in 2018 were 85 years or older (National Center for Health Statistics, 2022). Yet this corresponded only to less than 8% of the 2018 US population 85 or older.

More older people need care due to population aging, but they also have higher expectations for the quality of life as they age. Denmark has a universal care (social) system that cost 3.6% of GDP in 2019. Of this share of GDP, the spending on home long term care was 36% and on nursing home care 51% (OECD, 2021). This was possible because 57% of people 65 and over rated their health as good or very good (Regional Office for Europe, 2019). Older persons in Denmark have the right to participate in decision-making about their care and to receive personalized services. Relying on home care enables them to live as long as they want in their homes. The resulting system meets the needs of the country's high population share of older persons (20%) as well as the requirement for high efficiency.

News and Current Affairs

An important aspect of civic participation is familiarity with current events and news in order to be a knowledgeable citizen and informed voter. Differences in access and sources could result in inequitable civic participation.

In the United States, a survey of how respondents aged 65 years or over often got their news found that 68% said from television, 48% via a smart phone, computer or tablet, 25% from print publications and 21% from the radio (Shearer, 2021). In Sweden, based on national surveys between 2014 and 2018 on the use of traditional and digital consumption of news by people aged 66−85 years, there was concern that an age-based digital divide could affect democratic participation (Bergström, 2020). Though newspaper reading was declining, there was an increase in the reliance on digital newspapers. Radio and television use was stable.

Voting

Older citizens are more likely to be home owners and longtime residents of their communities, and they are often more connected to the political process (Hersh, 2020). The power of the 'Grey Vote' has been noted in close elections. In the United States, 75% of citizens aged 65 and older voted in the 2020 election, the best turnout of any age group (United States Census Bureau, 2021, Table 4c). In the United Kingdom, the turnout of those over 55 years was 83% compared to 58% for those under 55 years (Chrisp & Pearce, 2019). In Canada, this sense of civic involvement or duty was found to be more evident among older adults, who are more likely than younger citizens to vote in all levels of government elections. Voting rates among older voters has remained fairly stable and above the average (Table 3.2).

Public Office

A concern for future generations and a desire to make contributions to society can stimulate interest in political parties and elected office. Those with long careers as elected officials age in their jobs and others start a second career after retirement. No upper limit of age has been typically applied for elected posts. For example, in France, after 50 years as Mayor of Saint-Seurin-sur-l'Isle, M. Berthomé ran for re-election for the tenth time at age 98 but lost (Galiacy, 2021). The European Parliament has had members aged 88 and 89 years old (Oldest member (European Parliament), 2021). In Canada, appointed Senators can serve until age 75. In the United States, in the 118th Congress 74 members of the House of Representatives were aged 70 and over and the oldest representative was 86 years old (Stowe, 2023). In the United States Senate, 34 senators of 100 were 70 years or older. Two of the oldest members were 89 years old. The average age was 64 years.

Table 3.2 Older people tend to vote: Voter turnout by age, Canada, Federal elections, 2011, 2015 and 2019

Age groups	2019	2015	2011
Average all age groups	77%	77%	70%
18–24 years	68%	67%	55%
25–34 years	71%	70%	59%
35–44 years	75%	75%	65%
45–54 years	78%	79%	73%
55–64 years	81%	83%	80%
65–74 years	85%	86%	84%
75 years and older	79%	80%	79%

Source: Statistics Canada (2020b, Chart 1)

Political Activism

Many older people are active in organizations that either advocate for older people or for improving the conditions for people around the world. Such activism benefits the older person and improves their networks and also enables them to give back. There are international organizations such as HelpAge Global Network that support safe, healthy and dignified lives for older people worldwide. National organizations, such as the American Association of Retired Persons (AARP), actively advocate for older people and participate in political processes. The Elders, started in 2007 by Nelson Mandela, brings together independent older global leaders, such as Jimmy Carter, Gro Harlem Brundtland, Ban Ki-moon and Mary Robinson to work together for peace and human rights. Others build on personal interest and a desire to improve life and the health of the planet. Go Eco encourages older people to volunteer for humanitarian and wildlife conservation projects in Australia, Africa, and Central and South America. Local initiatives include grand parenting programs, growing food in gardens for food banks and tutoring children or migrants in English as a second language.

3.4 Social Construction of Aging and Increased Longevity Should Realistically Recognize Contributions in Later Life

Greater longevity is one of the greatest achievements of the modern era. However, because of significant social transformations that require social adaptations, recognition of the value of increased longevity is slow. There are two main reasons for this legacy thinking. First, it is based on partial estimates of the balance between contributions to and utilization of public services in later life. The dependency ratio, based on labour force participation, is used to argue this case. Second, the value of the contributions of the later life cohorts are underestimated. These entrenched ideas make it difficult to discard traditional views of old age and to reimagine an evolving phase of later life.

The aging process was viewed as an arc, where development in the early phases of life peaked in middle age and declined in older years. Aging is now understood as a human development process that is life affirming rather than life limiting. New thinking about aging is beginning to emerge. For example, ageivism refers to an ideology, which proposes social action for the protection and promotion of the rights of older people based on grounds of political, social and economic principles of identity, dignity and social justice (Doron, 2018).

The longer lifetime includes a progression of learning and growth resulting in continued human development. Later life is a period of multiple interrelated challenges, and older people are solution-multipliers in order to live life to the fullest. People in later life want to build a life of purpose until the end. Every extra day of life should be blessing as it adds to the period of self-actualization in the life course. The life course perspective recognizes that contributions can vary in content and intensity over the life span, and the totality can peak and ebb rather than progressively decline with age after early adulthood. With the varied human capital and experience built over a long lifetime, older people continue to contribute as active agents of change for society and future generations. The status that society accords to people in later life should reflect their lifetime of contributions to society. National policy responses based on the potential societal benefits from later life can enrich these extra years and thus enlarge the longevity dividend.

References

AARP & National Alliance for Caregiving. (2020, May). *Caregiving in the U.S. 2020* (Research report). https://www.caregiving.org/wp-content/uploads/2020/05/Full-Report-Caregiving-in-the-United-States-2020.pdf

AARP. (2022). *Global longevity economy outlook.* https://www.aarp.org/content/dam/aarp/research/surveys_statistics/econ/2022/global-longevity-economy-report.doi.10.26419-2Fint.00052.001.pdf

Arriagada, P. (2020). *The experiences and needs of older caregivers in Canada.* Statistics Canada, Insights on Canadian Society. https://www150.statcan.gc.ca/n1/pub/75-006-x/2020001/article/00007-eng.htm

Bergström, S. (2020). Exploring digital divides in older adults' news consumption. *Nordicom Review, 41*(2), 163–177. https://doi.org/10.2478/nor-2020-0021

Beznoska, M., & Hentze, T. (2017). Demographic change and income tax revenue in Germany: A microsimulation approach. *Public Sector Economics, 41*(1), 71–84. https://doi.org/10.3326/pse.41.1.8

Botham, R., & Graves, A. (2009). *The grey economy: How third age entrepreneurs are contributing to growth* (Research report). National Endowment for Science, Technology and the Arts (United Kingdom). https://media.nesta.org.uk/documents/the_grey_economy.pdf

Chrisp, J., & Pearce, N. (2019, May 21). *The rise of the grey vote.* IPR blog, University of Bath. https://blogs.bath.ac.uk/iprblog/2019/05/21/the-rise-of-the-grey-vote/

Cobb-Clark, D. A., & Gørgens, T. (2014). Parents' economic support of young-adult children: Do socioeconomic circumstances matter? *Journal of Population Economics, 27*(2), 447–471. https://doi.org/10.1007/s00148-013-0484-6

Davey, J. (2021, June 24). *More older New Zealanders are starting businesses—And they're motivated by more than just money.* The Conversation. https://theconversation.com/more-older-new-zealanders-are-starting-businesses-and-theyre-motivated-by-more-than-just-money-163003

Della Bosca, L. (2018, March 2). *Fear for the future of volunteers. Your life choices.* https://www.yourlifechoices.com.au/news/fear-for-the-future-of-volunteers/comment-page-2/

Department of Statistics. (2018, May). *What about seniors?* (No. 1). International Labour Organization, Spotlight on work statistics. https://ilo.org/wcmsp5/groups/public/%2D%2D-dgreports/%2D%2D-stat/documents/publication/wcms_629567.pdf

Doron, I. (2018). Re-thinking old age: Time for Ageivism. *Human Rights Defender, 27*(1), 33–36. https://papers.ssrn.com/sol3/papers.cfm?abstract_id=3195305

Drummond, D., Sinclair, D. & Bergen, R. (2020). *Ageing well* (White paper). Queen's University. https://www.queensu.ca/sps/sites/spswww/files/uploaded_files/publications/1%20Ageing%20Well%20Report%20-%20November%202020.pdf

European Commission. (2017, 16 August). *Growing the silver economy in Europe.* https://ec.europa.eu/digital-single-market/en/news/growing-silver-economy-europe

Fengler, W. (2021, January 14). *The silver economy is coming of age: A look at the growing spending power of seniors*. Brookings, Future Development. https://www.brookings.edu/blog/future-development/2021/01/14/the-silver-economy-is-coming-of-age-a-look-at-the-growing-spending-power-of-seniors/

Froats, P. (2011, September 16). *Chart: The ages of tax*. Canadian Business. https://www.canadianbusiness.com/blogs-and-comment/chart-the-ages-of-tax/

Fujioka, T. (2020, December 15). *Japan's $707 billion stimulus hinges on elderly spending money*. Bloomberg News Wire. https://www.bnnbloomberg.ca/japan-s-707-billion-stimulus-hinges-on-elderly-spending-money-1.1536957

Galiacy, J.-C. (2021, 2 February*). Âgé de 98 ans, il postulait à un dixième mandat consécutif dans cette commune de 3000 habitants* [At age 98, he stood for a tenth mandate in this community of 3,000 people]. Sud Ouest. https://www.sudouest.fr/gironde/saint-seurin-sur-l-isle/municipales-a-saint-seurin-sur-l-isle-33-marcel-berthome-plus-vieux-maire-de-france-battu-1178441.php

Goldman, D. P., Cutler, D., Rowe, J. W., Michaud, P.-C., Sullivan, J., Peneva, D., & Olshansky, S. J. (2013). Substantial health and economic returns from delayed aging may warrant a new focus for medical research. *Health Affairs, 32*(10), 1698–1705. https://doi.org/10.1377/hlthaff.2013.0052

Guberman, N., Lavoie, J.-P., Blein, L., & Olazabal, I. (2012). Baby boom caregivers: Care in the age of individualization. *The Gerontologist, 52*(2), 210–218. https://doi.org/10.1093/geront/gnr140

Hahmann, T., du Plessis, V., & Fournier-Savard, P. (2020). *Volunteering in Canada: Challenges and opportunities during the COVID-19 Pandemic*. Statistics Canada, STATCAN Covid-19: Data to Insights for a Better Canada. https://www150.statcan.gc.ca/n1/pub/45-28-0001/2020001/article/00037-eng.htm

Hersh, E. (2020). *Politics is for power. How to move beyond political hobbyism, take action, and make real change*. Scribner.

Howe, N. (2018, March 16). *The graying of wealth*. Forbes. https://www.forbes.com/sites/neilhowe/2018/03/16/the-graying-of-wealth/#1e4e53e4302d

Johnson, R. W., & Wang, C. X. (2019). The financial burden of paid home care on older adults: Oldest and sickest are least likely to have enough income. *Health Affairs, 38*(6), 994–1002. https://doi.org/10.1377/hlthaff.2019.00025

Kelly, J. (2019, October 26). *Millennials will become the richest generation in American history as baby boomers transfer over their wealth*. Forbes. https://www.forbes.com/sites/jackkelly/2019/10/26/millennials-will-become-richest-generation-in-american-history-as-baby-boomers-transfer-over-their-wealth/?sh=6c7ceb966c4b

Kibler, E., Wainwright, T., Kautonen, T., & Blackburn, R. (2015). Can social exclusion against 'older entrepreneurs' be managed? *Journal of Small Business Management, 53*(S1), 193–208. https://doi.org/10.1111/jsbm.12194

Laun, L, & Palme, M. (2017, September 19). *The recent rise of labour force participation of older workers in Sweden* (Working paper 2017:17). Institute for Evaluation of Labour Market and Education Policy. https://www.ifau.se/globalassets/pdf/se/2017/wp2017-17-the-recent-rise-of-labor-force-participation-of-older-workers-in-sweden.pdf

Levy, B. R., Slade, M. D., Kunkel, S. R., & Kasi, S. V. (2002). Longevity increased by positive self-perceptions of aging. *Journal of Personality and Social Psychology, 83*(2), 261–270. https://doi.org/10.1037/0022-3514.83.2.261

Living Assistance Services. (2019, February 1). *The shortage of personal support workers in Canada – Is there a solution?* Caring matters blog. https://www.laservices.ca/the-shortage-of-personal-support-workers-in-canada-is-there-a-solution/

Margolis, R. (2016). The changing demography of grandparenthood. *Journal of Marriage and Family, 78*(3), 610–622. https://doi.org/10.1111/jomf.12286

May, U., & Bauer, C. (2021). *Self-care in Europe: Economic and social impact on individuals and society.* Association of the European Self-Care Industry. https://aesgp.eu/content/uploads/2022/01/AESGP-Summary-Report-Self-Care-in-Europe-Economic-and-Social-Impact-on-Individuals-and-Society.pdf

McMahon, T. (2018, September 6). *Seniors and the generation spending gap*. Maclean's. https://www.macleans.ca/society/life/seniors-and-the-generation-spending-gap/
Mei, Z., Fast, J., & Eales, J. (2013, September 23). *Gifts of a lifetime: The contributions of older Canadians* (Final report). Seniors Association of Greater Edmonton. http://www.mysage.ca/public/download/documents/4754
Mtshali, M. N. G. (2016). Role reversal of rural black grandparents in South Africa. *Journal of Comparative Family Studies, 47*(3), 369–377. https://doi.org/10.3138/jcfs.47.3.369
National Center for Health Statistics. (2022). *Post-acute and long-term care providers and services users in the United States, 2017–2018*. Vital and Health Statistics, Series 3, Number 47. https://www.cdc.gov/nchs/data/series/sr_03/sr03-047.pdf
Nicol Economics. (2020). *Kinship care: The opportunity*. Report for Grandparents Plus (United Kingdom). https://kinship.org.uk/wp-content/uploads/Final_economic_case_text.pdf
OECD. (2020). *Who cares? Attracting and retaining care workers for the elderly*. OECD Health Policy Studies. OECD Publishing. https://www.oecd-ilibrary.org/social-issues-migration-health/who-cares-attracting-and-retaining-elderly-care-workers_92c0ef68-en
OECD. (2021). *Health at a glance 2021: OECD indicators*. OECD Publishing. https://www.oecd.org/health/health-at-a-glance/
Oldest member (European Parliament). (2021, February 14). In *Wikipedia*. https://en.wikipedia.org/wiki/Oldest_Member_(European_Parliament)
Regional Office for Europe. (2019). *Denmark: Country case study on the integrated delivery of long-term care*. World Health Organization. https://www.euro.who.int/__data/assets/pdf_file/0010/424648/Denmark-country-case-study-on-the-integrated.pdf
Research on Aging Policies and Practice. (2022, February 20). *Value of family caregiving in Canada* [Infographic]. University of Alberta and University of Manitoba. https://rapp.ualberta.ca/wp-content/uploads/sites/49/2022/02/Family-caregiving-worth-97-billion_2022-02-20.pdf
Revera and International Federation of Aging. (2012). *Revera report on ageism*. https://ifa.ngo/wp-content/uploads/2013/03/Revera-IFA-Ageism-Report.pdf
Revera. (2019). *Revera report on aging: Living a life of purpose*. https://reveraliving.com/en/think-with-us/reports-on-aging
Sandel, M. J. (2020). *The tyranny of merit: What's become of the common good?* Farrar, Straus and Giroux.
Schøtt, T., Rogoff, E., Herrington, M., & Kew, P. (2017). *GEM special report on senior entrepreneurship 2017*. Global Entrepreneurship Research Association. https://gemconsortium.org/report/gem-2016-2017-report-on-senior-entrepreneurship
Shearer, E. (2021, January 12). *More than eight-in-ten Americans get news from digital devices*. Pew Research Center. https://www.pewresearch.org/fact-tank/2021/01/12/more-than-eight-in-ten-americans-get-news-from-digital-devices/
Sinha, S., & Nolan, M. (2020, November). *Bringing long term care home*. National Institute on Aging (Canada). https://static1.squarespace.com/static/5c2fa7b03917eed9b5a436d8/t/5fb57afdbb4dec698ea3b7d2/1605729021992/BringLTCHome_V2.11.17%284%29pdf.pdf
Social Protection Department. (2014). *Social protection for older persons: Key policy trends and statistics* (Social protection policy paper No. 11). International Labour Organization. https://www.ilo.org/wcmsp5/groups/public/%2D%2D-dgreports/%2D%2D-dcomm/documents/publication/wcms_310211.pdf
Statistics Canada. (2017). *Working seniors in Canada*. Census in Brief. https://www12.statcan.gc.ca/census-recensement/2016/as-sa/98-200-x/2016027/98-200-x2016027-eng.cfm
Statistics Canada. (2019). *Family matters: Grandparents in Canada*. https://www150.statcan.gc.ca/n1/pub/11-627-m/11-627-m2019001-eng.htm
Statistics Canada. (2020a, November 24). *Almost one-quarter of Canadian seniors are caregivers*. The Daily. https://www150.statcan.gc.ca/n1/en/daily-quotidien/201124/dq201124a-eng.pdf?st=3f48pG9M

Statistics Canada. (2020b, February 26). *Reasons for not voting in the federal election, October 21, 2019.* The Daily. https://www150.statcan.gc.ca/n1/daily-quotidien/200226/dq200226b-eng.htm

Statistics Canada. (2021, February 11). *Diversity of charity and non-profit boards of directors: Overview of the Canadian non-profit sector.* The Daily. https://www150.statcan.gc.ca/n1/daily-quotidien/210211/dq210211a-eng.htm

Statistics Canada. (2022a). *A portrait of Canada's growing population aged 85 and older from the 2021 Census.* Census in Brief. https://www12.statcan.gc.ca/census-recensement/2021/as-sa/98-200-X/2021004/98-200-X2021004-eng.pdf

Statistics Canada. (2022c, April 12). *Charitable donors, 2020.* The Daily. https://www150.statcan.gc.ca/n1/en/daily-quotidien/220412/dq220412d-eng.pdf?st=TEDuh5hS

Statistics of Income Division. (2023). *Basic Tables Part 3: Tax Computation.* Internal Revenue Service (USA). https://www.irs.gov/statistics/soi-tax-stats-individual-income-tax-returns-complete-report-publication-1304-basic-tables-part-3

Stowe, L. (2023, February 6). *How old is the 118th Congress?* FiscalNote blog. https://fiscalnote.com/blog/how-old-118th-congress

Terrell, K. (2019, December 19). *Americans 50 and older would be world's third largest economy, AARP study finds.* AARP Advocacy. https://www.aarp.org/politics-society/advocacy/info-2019/older-americans-economic-impact-growth.html

The age of the grandparent has arrived. (2023, January 12). *The Economist.* https://www.economist.com/international/2023/01/12/the-age-of-the-grandparent-has-arrived

Toossi, M., & Torpey, E. (2017, May). *Older workers: Labour force trends and career options.* United States Bureau of Labor Statistics, Career Outlook. https://www.bls.gov/careeroutlook/2017/article/older-workers.htm

United States Census Bureau. (2021). *Voting and Registration Tables. Voting and Registration in the Election of November 2020.* https://www.census.gov/topics/public-sector/voting/data/tables.html

Vanier Institute of the Family. (2019, February 8). *In Focus 2019: Grandparents in Canada.* https://vanierinstitute.ca/in-focus-2019-grandparents-in-canada/

Zimmer, Z., & Treleaven, E. (2020). The rise and prominence of skip-generation households in lower- and middle-income countries. *Population and Development Review, 46*(4), 709–733. https://onlinelibrary.wiley.com/doi/abs/10.1111/padr.12349

Chapter 4
Long Life Learning

4.1 Evolutionary Roots of Learning

Learning started as a primal instinct, closely allied with survival. From an evolutionary perspective, the human brain evolved to do better at living by learning throughout life (OECD, 2002). The brain is always learning. As a consequence, individuals are a result of their learning (Jarvis, 1987) and varied because of their individual learning. Those that learned to change and adapt succeeded in the process of natural selection. Learning is a fundamental stimulus to life and without it humans could never transcend their biology and function effectively as social beings or as a community. Learning is essential to our humanity (Jarvis, 2006).

Biological, emotional, social and cognitive motivations activate learning behaviour, which starts in babies and lasts through life. Though not used equally frequently or equally well, almost all motivations are driven by curiosity, inquiry, interest and need to know. Humans evolved to learn. Lifelong learning therefore has evolutionary origins.

For species survival, humans became social. While genetic heritage helped develop individuals, learned knowledge held by groups became the repository of culture, which was transmitted through generations. As the environment and conditions of life changed, both individual learning and the stock of societal learning grew in importance. Learning enabled adaptions to the environment. It also enabled sufficient understanding of the environment to change it and to improve life for those living in it through social or behavioural innovation. Since the conditions of the world and life experiences are unpredictable, a person is always learning from novel situational and environmental information, which adds to the stock of human capital. Evolution has thus proven through the centuries that learning is important for individual development and successful communities. Oral transmission soon became insufficient.

S. Brink, *The Longevity Dividend*, International Perspectives on Aging 39,
https://doi.org/10.1007/978-3-031-35335-2_4

As the importance of knowledge grew for society, the transmission of consolidated knowledge and skills became formalized through formal education from childhood. Schooling provided basic education, which is the foundation upon which further knowledge and skills are accumulated. Higher education offered specialized professional and technical knowledge. Working age people learned work skills and technical knowledge through training and work place learning. However, life continues beyond the working years, and continuous learning is therefore required to respond to the demands of later life and to the changing environment.

4.2 The Contemporary Stimuli for Learning Through Life

The need to learn is affected by changes that occur in a lifetime. Just a scant two decades ago, centenarians were rare, there were no robots with artificial intelligence, no one had a smart phone and catastrophic climate events were less common. Yet these are every day occurrences for everyone living in this century regardless of age. Multiple simultaneous changes results in living in periods of ambiguity. So, to succeed in life, given an average lifespan of 85 years, an individual is driven to adapt at a pace commensurate with changes in external factors. The drivers for change in contemporary society arise in a variety of life domains, which are themselves changing at different speeds. Table 4.1 provides some examples.

Table 4.1 Changes occurring in selected domains that require appropriate responses for successful aging

Change driver	Increasing life span	Knowledge generation	Technology	Climate change
Projected change	More children born since 2000 are likely to live 100 years (Christensen et al., 2009)	In 1900, knowledge doubled approximately every 100 years; since 2020, knowledge doubles every 12 months. At the same time, the useful lifespan of knowledge is decreasing (Fuller, 1981)	Technological change is accelerating exponentially (Kurzweil, 2005). Changes can be disruptive	The rate of change in climate over the next century will be at least 10 times quicker than any climate shift in the past 65 million years (Diffenbaugh & Field, 2013)
Pace of change	Relatively slow	Fast and complex	Very fast and complex	Peaking in this century
Predictability	Predictable	Predictable speed but unpredictable new knowledge	Predictable growth but unpredictable products and services	Predictable climate events but not the time and place of storms and fires

Author's elaboration, 2023

4.3 Learning and Life Are Interdependent

In earlier times, it was possible to dedicate the early years of one's life to learning and this provided a sufficient base for the rest of life. Traditional knowledge was sufficient and was passed on to younger generations. People did not live as long or experience dramatic changes in life events, context or environment. Even so they continued to learn through life informally from experience and from each other. Now, if life lasts nearly a century, 12 years of learning or even more in early life cannot prepare individuals for the demands of life in the remaining 60 years or more. Learning and life are interdependent. The more knowledge that is acquired, the more resilient an individual becomes in the face of change. Continuous learning is a relevant means to prepare for contingencies in an unknown future.

The concept of 'half-life of knowledge' explains the duration of the accuracy and utility of facts and information from the time they are learned. The half-life of knowledge is the amount of time that has to elapse before half of the knowledge is superseded or shown to be untrue. Much of knowledge has a predictable expiry date based on the degree of specificity and specialization (Arbesman, 2013; Schüppel, 1997).

About half the knowledge acquired in school or university, especially foundational and generic knowledge, deteriorates slowly and lasts for 20 years or more. In contrast, specialized knowledge, for example related to medicine, is valid for a shorter time (Schüppel, 1997). The speed of technological evolution makes information technology knowledge outmoded very quickly. A century ago, an engineer's knowledge gained at university was estimated to lose half its relevance in about 35 years, but this interval had by 1960 already fallen to 10 years (Charette, 2013). For an engineer to stay up to date with professional knowledge if the half-life of engineering knowledge was ten years, learning would be required for 5 hours a week during 48 weeks a year (Jones, 1966).

4.4 Learning Through Life

The need for learning depends on the interaction of two factors: age-appropriate knowledge and the context in which life is lived. The life course theory notes that an individual's life experience depends on contextual factors such as life span development, human agency, historical time, and geographical place (Elder et al., 2003). Therefore, the longer one lives, the person's lived experience becomes more and more diverse and requires both generic and specific knowledge and skills for quality of life and contribution to society. Learning skills are desirable and they can be improved with time so knowledge can be cumulatively gained over the lifetime. Learning skills require unlearning of useless information (disconnected telephone numbers, for instance), upskilling (electronic filing of taxes) or the learning of totally new information (such as Telehealth services or new financial saving instruments).

As individuals progress through life, their needs for knowledge and skills change depending on life events and living environment as well as the progress of world history. The demand for life-related content can change through life, though some needs could remain constant. For example, all ages may need to understand how to use a smart phone, but many in later life would be more interested in better understanding how 'power of attorney' works. The ways to gain access to learning remain the same, though individuals choose those that work best for themselves as they grow older.

4.5 Is a Prolongation of Adult Learning Approaches Effective in Later Life?

Lifelong learning is sometimes considered synonymous with adult learning. Essentially, since all learning beyond initial learning occurs in adulthood, adult learning is assumed to serve all ages beyond youth until death. It implies that adult learning is the culmination of lifelong learning and is sufficient for the years beyond retirement. This idea assumes that learning needs in the later years are the same as in the working years. This is questionable. Table 4.2 identifies the differences in current practice.

Is it just a question of terminology? Older adults do participate in some adult learning. It is therefore tempting to add a sub-section for later life learning to the adult learning discipline, which is already better developed and more generously funded. However, despite some overlaps, there are considerable differences between the needs of adults and older people. The demand for the learning that matters is different at the two stages and the provision of learning is also different. The pedagogy would require scaling older and scaling wider, since learners can range from 25 to over 90 with different needs and capacities. One view might be that this would not serve either learner clientele well. An alternate view might be that the relationship between adult learning and later life learning is similar to the relationship between early childhood learning and formal schooling. Although early childhood learning and formal schooling are linked and benefit from continuity, they differ enough in developing opportunities and delivery to be seen as separate disciplines.

The simple extension of adult learning until death underestimates the value of lifelong learning. It also undersells the need for learning in later life. Lifelong learning subsumes adult learning. For purposes of organization, the provision of hard and soft learning infrastructure could be targeted by age (preschooling) or stage of life. However, lifelong learning is not segmented into such chunks but rather it is a continuous process. There are overlaps. For instance, learning through play can extend throughout life, and learning to meet the demands of the labour market can occur in the working years and extend to 'working retirement'. If adult learning dominates

Table 4.2 Differences between adult learning and late-life learning in current practice

Adult learning in current practice	Learning beyond the working years
Learners	
Adults in their peak working years	Late-life learners in their post-retirement years
Motivated by career-related goals	Motivated by life challenges, personal interest, need for intellectual stimulation or improvement to their quality of life
Often able to access financial aid and support (e.g., counselling)	Generally personal investment of time, effort and funds
Courses and topics	
Job related knowledge and skills, upskilling, reskilling; vocational, occupational and professional, specialized subjects	Short, intermittent courses; currently many are offered for recreation and entertainment; much self-learning
Wide choice	Based on demand
Credit or credentials	No assessment or credentials
Learning provision	
Known stakeholders	No stakeholders
Formal, internships, online	Formal, informal or online
Universities and colleges, professional institutions, unions	Universities (third age) and colleges, community centres, retirement communities
Financial incentives	No financial incentives
Government or corporate investment, justified because of private and public/corporate returns	Generally inadequately funded, dependent on fees

Author's elaboration, 2023

lifelong learning in the public discourse, there is a danger that learning in later years remains under-developed or, worse, that learning ends at retirement so that the pursuit of life potential is terminated prematurely.

4.6 Learning for Life After Work

Retirement was considered a rite of passage into old age, when one ceased to be in the labour force. When the period between exit from work and death was fairly short, it was assumed that it was a period of slowing down, withdrawal and decline. It was expected that older people would fill their time with activities they were too busy to pursue while working, such as philosophical reflection on the meaning of life, contemplating achievements and readying oneself for death (Formosa, 2014). This was a continuation of Erikson's theory that competences were acquired in all previous stages, but the ninth stage (added by his wife) was dominated by despair and low self-esteem due to the experience of deteriorating body and mind (Erikson & Erikson, 1998). Lately, the variety of learning options has increased. However, they tend to focus on leisure, recreation and special interests, or adult learning of this type is simply extended to the older population. Even training or preparation for being retired from employment has been cursory. With retirement lasting perhaps a couple of decades, even a three-day retirement course would be inadequate preparation for this phase of life.

Attempts to increase learning by older adults have a long history (Glendenning, 1989). In the seventies, the disciplines of Geragogy and educational gerontology were created, with a focus on the teaching of older adults and learning in later life. Two of the objectives were to inform older adults and modify their behaviours, on the one hand, and to educate the public to improve attitudes towards older people, on the other (Peterson, 1976). At that time, the life expectancy was shorter, however, and the number of years in retirement were fewer. There was a tendency to draw on the existing systems of provision of learning for older adults. This tended to treat education as a place or an activity rather than in terms of yielding results for the learner. Little importance was given to the evolving needs of long-lived older people, their previous diverse learning trajectories or the heterogeneity in learning capacities in the last decades of life.

Learning for, and learning by, older adults is evolving but far more slowly than the speed at which the population is aging. While some opportunities for healthy aging are available, the majority of this large population segment is underserved. Since a long later life is a new phenomenon, it is time to completely rethink learning in later life.

4.7 Better Understanding of Later Life and the Role of Learning

Since the aging of the population is unprecedented, the substantial increases in the number of older persons and their proportion in the population have been perceived as a challenge to society. Though the growth in the older population was anticipated, the implications of its interaction with longevity took longer to understand. The differences in the aging experience led to a re-examination of the life course.

The first insight was that conditions in each stage, such as childhood, could affect the outcomes over the lifetime, especially if they occurred during a critical period of development. Further refinement led to consideration of timing, length of exposure and the importance of life events that had delayed but lasting consequences for development and that affected future outcomes and potential responses. This led to consideration of accumulated assets and chains of risks that are acquired over time and which shape later outcomes. The next step was to consider a person's agency in altering the trajectory to more positive outcomes than those predicted by their assets, risks and antecedents (Berkman et al., 2011; Elder et al., 2003; Hendricks, 2012). Consideration of the role of learning in making choices to improve outcomes came even later.

The drive to make the longer aging process positive and to improve the outcomes for people and societies led to research about normal aging. The concept of 'successful aging' was developed in the 1980s (Rowe & Kahn, 1987). It tended to be a medical view, where success was defined as 'a non-pathological state', focusing on three main components: low probability of disease and disease-related disability, high cognitive and functional capacity, and active engagement with life (Rowe & Kahn, 1997). Later research has shown that learning is a key strategy for productive aging (Stowe & Conney, 2015). Though easily related to work, learning during later life allows people to maximize the positive aspects of aging by mobilizing their productive potential, given their own constraints and opportunities (Butler & Gleason, 1985). Caro et al. (1993) suggested that productive aging is the capacity of older individuals to engage in paid or unpaid activities that result in useful goods or services. These goods and services can improve one's own life and the society in which they live. A broader view of productive aging suggested engaging with the positive aspects of growing older, undertaking meaningful activities in later life and making one's own life better while contributing to society (Schulte et al., 2018). Productive aging included a life span approach, leading to an integrated well-rounded life with mutually valuable contributions to self and society within a supportive multigenerational culture. Research has confirmed that learning is a key strategy for this latter view of productive aging.

4.8 Learning in Later Life

Later life is the ultimate step in human development. Since one only lives once, it makes sense to make life the best it can be until the end. The power of learning improves the possibility of achieving that goal.

The idea that learning is not required in later life, because all previously learned knowledge is sufficient and cognitive declines will make further learning difficult, reveals serious misperceptions. Age is no barrier to learning. The reason for any cognitive declines may be that learning has ceased, which thus leads to more deterioration in quality of life.

What matters now is 'long life learning'. Since an individual has no personal experience with aging or prolonged life, the worthwhile knowledge and behaviours have to be learned in order to face extended life with confidence. To thrive, each person has to adapt to the challenges of life in the later years in relation to one's personal capacities. This means continuing to build human capital, but also correcting and updating knowledge and experience to confront the demands of a changing world. Learning enables a person to utilize existing and new knowledge for critical thinking and problem solving, which facilitates coping successfully with new and unpredictable issues of life and taking advantage of opportunities. Learning yields two outcomes. One is to support the process of 'becoming' (Hodkinson et al., 2008) or to achieve one's life potential. The other is to achieve a productive life by making the best use of the later years.

Learning also makes knowledge work possible in later life. Late-life learners use higher order knowledge and skills in today's knowledge economy (Bloom et al., 1956). Knowledge workers can apply current knowledge in new ways in novel situations and generate new knowledge. They can make wise decisions about consumption because they understand the knowledge and technology embedded in modern products and services. This creates more potential for experiencing quality of life than in earlier generations.

The sequence of experiences in one's life-world creates an individual learning biography that results in a personal repository of knowledge. Lifelong learning offers a perspective of one's own life trajectory and the ways in which desirable changes could be achieved in a lifelong process. An individual provided with timely knowledge can manipulate the available levers to influence the pathways of development throughout life. The outcomes of lifelong learning are only as strong as the weakest link in the trajectory. At present, these outcomes are more easily achieved earlier in the life course than in later life because later life is not well served with learning opportunities.

4.9 Lifelong Learning in Later Life and Its Private and Public Benefits

Would returns to learning in later life be worth the investment? Would society face higher costs without learning in later life? The costs of learning in the later years currently are not as high as for other ages, and most learners self-fund their efforts. Since learning is a private as well as a public good, it is worthwhile examining the value of promoting learning in later life.

4.10 Private Benefits from Learning for Individuals in Later Life

Continuously increasing the value of their personal human capital allows individuals to reach their potential. By providing assurance based on knowledge and confidence in action, it increases success in later life. Individuals are able to tailor their learning so that they can improve their quality of life commensurate with their capacities. They are also able to contribute to their families, communities and the world they live in by playing the roles expected of them well. Because learning helps them to manage their health and their capacities, they can experience life satisfaction and fulfillment.

The returns from autonomy and independence are valuable for individuals and their families. Their costs for health and personal care may be higher in later years, but with learned healthy behaviours and self-care, most people's years of good health are prolonged.

4.11 Public Benefits from Learning in Later Life for Society

Learning increases skills and competencies and augments their societal value in three ways: absolute, relative and average (OECD & CERI, 2007). This can be applied to late-life learning. Learning enhances competencies for productive individuals. In the broadest sense it enables a person's proficient performance in all social roles – worker, caregiver, citizen and consumer. Therefore, it would be natural to promote lifelong learning until the end of life.

4.11.1 Absolute Measure of Competencies and Later Learners

The higher the number of people who have high competencies, the greater the benefit both for those individuals and for society. In developed countries, the individuals in any given proportion of the population 70 and over are more educated than in earlier generations and can be a productive segment of the population. They contribute to their communities through paid work, unpaid work, volunteering and wise consumption. Such societies offer more opportunities to individuals and have greater capacity for receiving their contributions.

4.11.2 Relative Measure of Competencies and Later Learners

Individuals or societies enjoy a comparative advantage if they have greater competencies than other individuals or societies. A large proportion of those in their later years have specialized or have life experiences that make them a 'cognitive reserve' for their communities. Older people in the labour force can offset shortages due to a shrinking workforce of younger people. In addition, they can serve on committees, on boards, as advisors, as mentors or as entrepreneurs. Societies are able to manage the resources and contributions of older people for maximum benefit.

4.11.3 Average National Competencies

Individuals can benefit more if they live in a country with high average competencies than if they do not. Competencies possessed collectively in a population represents national human capital, a major asset that countries can harness to achieve national goals for a desired future. There are greater opportunities, more resources and better collaboration. In developed countries the population in later life could compose almost a fifth to a quarter of the population, so their human capital is significant. Without learning, people in later life could lower the average national competencies, creating a drag on progress. Learning in this life stage can increase the human capital of the large later life segment of the population. This can, for example, speed up technology adoption, implement public action for climate change and increase investment in innovative enterprises. Older generations transmit their stock of learning to younger and future generations. Because learning helps to level the playing field, it reduces the human capital gap between generations. Without learning this gap will grow and reinforce the inequalities in society. Learning throughout life is a knowledge equalizer over time.

4.12 Lifelong Learning Incorporates Learning into Living

Lifelong learning has been discussed for decades. No standard definition of lifelong learning exists that is accepted worldwide, although several versions have been proposed in order to operationalize the concept. Specific understanding and even interpretations of the term vary widely around the world, and there is no agreement on what exactly lifelong learning means (UNESCO Institute for Lifelong Learning [UIL], 2016). In addition to causing confusion, this hinders the development of policies or implementation strategies (Bengtsson, 2013). The term may work better in practice than in theory.

In most parts of the world, support for lifelong learning is strong because of its relationship to personal and professional development. It is generally accepted that lifelong learning is a goal oriented, intentional activity which results in multiple long-term benefits. Such a process is often related to knowledge, skills and competencies that improve function, performance and contribution in several domains. For example, skills and competencies can improve personal, social and civic outcomes (Commission of the European Communities, 2000).

Most definitions of lifelong learning describe learning throughout life. There is, however, little clarity about the mechanisms that provide lifelong learning for the population of every age. As individuals develop through life, they continue individually to complete their own stock of human capital using different means of learning according to their needs and opportunities. While some definitions mention purposeful learning activity, some only suggest that learning can be acquired in different ways. Others specifically list formal, non-formal and informal learning and even online learning.

A generally accepted cluster of ideas that are related to lifelong learning suggests nonetheless that it is an umbrella concept. Table 4.3 incorporates selected terms and components that are commonly associated with lifelong learning.

Lifelong learning has tended to be condensed according to whatever supply system was in place. Earlier the formal education system was designed as initial, adult and continuing education to support a life course that could be described as 'learn-do-retire'. It was only in the 1970s that lifelong learning included concepts that emphasized learning, rather than education, in an integrated system of provision

Table 4.3 Lifelong learning is an umbrella concept

Lifelong learning (subsumes permanent, recurrent and continuous learning)					
Life course	Life wide, life deep	Modes of learning	Learning aids	Duration	Results
Birth Infancy Childhood Young adulthood Working age Old age Death	Formal or informal Learning abroad Real life context Authentic Experience Personal	Formal/non formal Informal On-line Self-directed Professional or specialized Internship Apprenticeship Multi-disciplinary	Teachers Peers, co-learners Inter- or multi-generational Learning materials (texts, presentations, tables, figures, audio-visual, etc.)	Years, sequential Short-term, intermittent months, weeks or days Long period of trial and error Split, gap between stimulus and insight	Cumulative Human capital Changed behaviours Adaptation and growth Transformation

Author's elaboration, 2023

with pathways between its inter-related elements (International Labour Organization [ILO], 2019). Fifty years later, the idea of lifelong learning continues to evolve.

4.13 Societal Losses If Lifelong Learning Does Not Extend Through Life

Lifelong learning implies that learning is a lifetime activity and that it uses opportunities for learning that are equitably available at all life stages. It is important for people to enjoy a productive life course, and undervaluing this can have long term consequences (Agronin, 2014). Overlooking learning in later life would result in the loss of many of the benefits that flow to society from longevity. The economic and social costs of inequity in lifelong learning are high for both individuals and society.

If lifelong learning is poorly designed for the needs of later life, or if learning is completely excluded, people's human capital would decline over their lifetime because information is outdated and new information and skills are lacking. People would be unprepared to meet the demands of a changing world as they age. This would reduce their quality of life and life satisfaction as they would be unable to reach their full potential or contribute to society.

The national human capital amounts to about 65% of the wealth of high-income countries (World Bank, 2017). Society would incur a sizeable reduction in national wealth if the contribution to national human capital that a fifth or more of the population makes is sub-optimal. The national economy would not grow as much as it could if the contributions by the entire population are optimal. If the average time spent in education (assuming average learning) by a population rises by one year, then economic output per head of the population could grow by between 4% and 6% in the long run (Spitzer, 2006). The distribution of lifelong learning would be incomplete if late-life learning is excluded, in which case countries would knowingly forgo economic growth.

Neglecting late-life learning would impose high social costs on society, too. Because some people in later life will have lower health outcomes and function poorly, they are likely to consume more public services. A more unequal society will result since the learning generations would function relatively better. This would result in the older population being undervalued and marginalized. Inequities could cause polarization among generations. Moreover, society would face higher public social spending for the older generation because more people would be less autonomous. This would be the opposite of a society that benefits from the contributions by the majority of older people. The younger generations would need to shoulder the costs of such dependency. These negative consequences for later life and working generations and for society as a whole would be a signal of maladaptation to population aging.

4.14 Growing Support for Learning as a Right of Citizenship

During the last several decades evidence has mounted on the value of lifelong learning for people, the economy and society. This made it necessary to shift to a lifelong learning culture and a learning society (OECD & CERI, 2000). A Learning Society is one where individuals and society use knowledge for both economic growth and social advancement. The pressure was growing to change the narrative for both supply of and demand for learning. Societies and governments would first develop a vision for systematically shaping a desirable future through learning. Countries would ensure that learning opportunities would be commensurate with the demands of a changing world. At the same time, individuals would be motivated by a mindset of continuous learning and would engage in lifelong learning as a normal part of life.

These ideas about the role of lifelong learning have begun to be codified to support personal growth, economic prosperity and social equity. The UN Universal Declaration of Human Rights (United Nations, 1948) recognizes the right to education as a human right and states that education shall be directed to the full development of the human personality (Article 26). The International Covenant on Economic, Social and Cultural Rights (United Nations, 1966) establishes that education shall enable all persons to participate effectively in a free society (Article 13.1). The Committee on Economic, Social, and Cultural Rights (United Nations, 1999) recognized that education is a means of realizing other human rights. Although later life learning is not explicit in these statements, words such as full and all ensure that the statements encompass both later life and lifelong learning.

As the realization of the importance of lifelong learning spread, more governments and other organizations began to take steps in this regard. In the United

Kingdom, the Inquiry into the future of lifelong learning links the right to learn throughout life to benefits to the individual, such as freedom of choice and dignity, and to benefits to society, which gains prosperity and democratic function (Schuller & Watson, 2009). In the United Kingdom, the culture of lifelong learning has been described as a nationwide culture that would ensure learning for everyone from birth to the end of life (Fryer, 1997).

In 2020, the report 'Embracing a culture of lifelong learning' of the UNESCO Institute of Lifelong Learning promoted the idea of learning through life as a human right and a responsibility of citizenship (UIL, 2020). Since lifelong learning has served as an auxiliary system rather than as a central organizing principle, it argued, reconceptualizing the lifelong learning ecosystem would be important. This system would have supporting legal frameworks, where learners can pursue a variety of pathways along their life course in order to achieve their full potential and provide their value to society.

4.15 Lifelong Learning Is a Shared Responsibility

Learning is a mutual responsibility and a collective obligation. Learning is also an individual responsibility, regardless of age, for more than personal benefit. Through learning, the knowledge accumulated and created serves as a public good to improve life for all. This responsibility is shared with society and the state because of the benefits experienced by past, present and future generations. The shared responsibilities for lifelong learning in later life are described below.

4.15.1 Individual

Learning is voluntary, self-directed and could be self-funded. Continuous and lifelong learning is necessary to manage the demands of life. It is linked to the obligation to acquire knowledge and share it with others and to contribute to society.

4.15.2 Society

Many actors and stakeholders are involved in learning. They direct, support or participate in learning for lifelong human development, including for late-life learners. Their involvement varies from organizing formal and non-formal courses in person or online, managing delivery, designing resources and teaching.

4.15.3 *The State*

In order to raise the level of learning of the population as a whole, the state provides leadership and assists implementation through policies, regulations and financing. Governments are responsible to ensure the equity and efficiency of options for learning for all citizens throughout life.

4.16 The Right to Lifelong Learning is Not Age-Limited

With some exceptions, people can learn almost anything at any age. Learning in later life is an integral part of lifelong learning. The right to learning does not have age limits. The lack of opportunities for learning to meet the needs of later life is not only a policy failure – it can also be an abdication of civic responsibility. For equity, investment in learning at any age should provide the same opportunities and assign the same value to the intended outcomes. However, universal entitlement to learning is only of value if it is accessed and used by everyone of all ages. Lifelong learning will remain the responsibility of the individual, but it is shared with society's institutions within a culture of learning that assures wellbeing and positive human development to all people of all ages.

References

Agronin, M. E. (2014). From Cicero to Cohen: Developmental theories of aging, from antiquity to the present. *The Gerontologist, 54*(1), 30–39. https://doi.org/10.1093/geront/gnt032

Arbesman, S. (2013). *The half-life of facts: Why everything we know has an expiration date.* Penguin.

Bengtsson, J. (2013). National strategies for implementing lifelong learning (LLL) – The gap between policy and reality: An international perspective. *International Review of Education, 59*(3), 343–352. https://www.jstor.org/stable/24637133

Berkman, L. F., Ertel, K. A., & Glymour, M. M. (2011). Aging and social intervention: Life course perspectives. In R. H. Binstock & L. K. George (Eds.), *Handbook of aging and the social sciences* (7th ed., pp. 337–351). Elsevier.

Bloom, B. S., Engelhart, M. D., Furst, E. J., Hill, W. H., & Krathwohl, D. R. (1956). *Taxonomy of educational objectives: The classification of educational goals (Handbook I: Cognitive domain).* David McKay.

Butler, R. N., & Gleason, H. P. (1985). *Productive aging: Enhancing vitality in later life.* Springer.

Caro, F. G., Bass, S. A., & Chen, Y.-P. (1993). Introduction: Achieving a productive aging society. In S. A. Bass, F. G. Caro, & Y.-P. Chen (Eds.), *Achieving a productive aging society* (pp. 3–25) Auburn House.

Charette, R. N. (2013, September 4). *An engineering career: Only a young person's game?* IEEE Spectrum https://spectrum.ieee.org/an-engineering-career-only-a-young-persons-game

Christensen, K., Doblhammer, G., Rau, R., & Vaupel, J. W. (2009). Ageing populations: The challenges ahead. *Lancet, 374*(3696), 1196–1208. https://doi.org/10.1016/S0140-6736(09)61460-4

Commission of the European Communities. (2000). *A memorandum on lifelong learning* (SEC(2000) 1832) [Working paper]. https://uil.unesco.org/i/doc/lifelong-learning/policies/european-communities-a-memorandum-on-lifelong-learning.pdf

Elder, G. H., Jr., Johnson, M. K., & Crosnoe, R. (2003). The emergence and development of life course theory. In J. T. Mortimer & M. J. Shanahan (Eds.), *Handbook of the life course* (pp. 3–19). Springer. https://doi.org/10.1007/978-0-306-48247-2_1

Erikson, E. H., & Erikson, J. (1998). *The life cycle completed: Extended version with new chapters on the ninth stage of development*. W.W. Norton.

Diffenbaugh, N. S., & Field, C. B. (2013). Changes in ecologically critical terrestrial climate conditions. *Science, 341*(6145), 486–492. https://doi.org/10.1126/science.1237123

Formosa, M. (2014). Lifelong learning in later life. In B. Schmidt-Hertha, S. J. Krašovec, & M. Formosa (Eds.), *Learning across generations in Europe: Contemporary issues in older adult education* (pp. 11–21). Sense Publishers. https://doi.org/10.1007/978-94-6209-902-9_2

Fryer, R. H. (1997). *Learning for the 21st century: First report of the national advisory group for continuing education and lifelong learning*. National Advisory Group for Continuing Education and Lifelong Learning (NAGCELL). https://www.voced.edu.au/content/ngv%3A35226

Fuller, R. B. (1981). *Critical path*. St. Martin's Griffin.

Glendenning, F. (1989). Educational gerontology in Britain as an emerging field of study and practice. *Educational Gerontology, 15*(2), 121–131. https://doi.org/10.1080/0380127890150202

Hendricks, J. (2012). Considering life course concepts. *The Journals of Gerontology, Series B: Psychological Sciences and Social Sciences, 67*(2), 226–231. https://doi.org/10.1093/geronb/gbr147

Hodkinson, P., Ford, G., Hodkinson, H., & Hawthorn, R. (2008). Retirement as a learning process. *Educational Gerontology, 34*(3), 167–184. https://doi.org/10.1080/03601270701835825

International Labour Organization. (2019). *Lifelong learning: Concepts, issues and actions*. https://www.ilo.org/wcmsp5/groups/public/%2D%2D-ed_emp/%2D%2D-ifp_skills/documents/publication/wcms_711842.pdf

Jarvis, P. (1987). *Adult learning in the social context*. Croom Helm.

Jarvis, P. (2006). *Towards a comprehensive theory of human learning*. Routledge.

Jones, T. F. (1966). The dollars and sense of continuing education. *IEEE Transactions on Aerospace and Electronic Systems, AES-2*(2), 140–142. https://ieeexplore.ieee.org/document/4501735

Kurzweil, R. (2005). *The singularity is near: When humans transcend biology*. Penguin.

OECD. (2002). *Understanding the brain: Towards a new learning science*. https://www.oecd-ilibrary.org/education/understanding-the-brain_9789264174986-en

OECD & Centre for Educational Research and Innovation. (2000). *Knowledge management in the learning society*. https://www.oecd-ilibrary.org/education/knowledge-management-in-the-learning-society_9789264181045-en

OECD & Centre for Educational Research and Innovation. (2007). *Understanding the social outcomes of learning*. https://www.oecd.org/education/ceri/understandingthesocialoutcomesoflearning.htm

Peterson, D. A. (1976). Educational gerontology: The state of the art. *Educational Gerontology, 1*(1), 61–73. https://doi.org/10.1080/03601277.1976.12049517

Rowe, J. W., & Kahn, R. L. (1987). Human aging: Usual and successful. *Science, 237*(4811), 143–149. https://doi.org/10.1126/science.3299702

Rowe, J. W., & Kahn, R. L. (1997). Successful aging. *The Gerontologist, 37*(4), 433–440. https://doi.org/10.1093/geront/37.4.433

Schuller, T., & Watson, D. (2009). *Learning through life: Inquiry into the future for lifelong learning (summary)*. National Institute of Adult Continuing Education. https://www.cmv-educare.com/wp-content/uploads/2015/12/schuller.pdf

Schulte, P. A., Grosch, J., Scholl, J. C., & Tamers, S. L. (2018). Framework for considering productive aging and work. *Journal of Occupational and Environmental Medicine, 60*(5), 440–448. https://www.ncbi.nlm.nih.gov/pmc/articles/PMC6262835/

Schüppel, J. (1997). *Wissensmanagement. Organisatorisches Lernen im Spannungsfeld von Wissens- und Lernbarrieren* [Knowledge management. Organizational learning in the field of tension between knowledge and learning barriers]. Gabler.

Spitzer, M. (2006). Brain research and learning over the life cycle. In *Personalizing education* (Centre for Educational Research and Innovation.) (pp. 47–62). OECD Publishing. https://doi.org/10.1787/9789264036604-4-en

Stowe, J. D., & Cooney, T. M. (2015). Examining Rowe and Kahn's concept of successful aging: Importance of taking a life course perspective. *The Gerontologist, 55*(1), 43–50. https://pubmed.ncbi.nlm.nih.gov/24906516/

UNESCO Institute for Lifelong Learning. (2016). *3rd global report on adult learning and education: The impact of adult learning and education on health and well-being, employment and the labour market, and social, civic and community life*. https://unesdoc.unesco.org/ark:/48223/pf0000245913

UNESCO Institute for Lifelong Learning. (2020). *Embracing a culture of lifelong learning: Contribution to the futures of education initiative*. https://uil.unesco.org/lifelong-learning/embracing-culture-lifelong-learning

United Nations. (1948). *Universal declaration of human rights*. https://www.un.org/en/about-us/universal-declaration-of-human-rights

United Nations. (1966). *International covenant on economic, social and cultural rights*. https://www.ohchr.org/en/instruments-mechanisms/instruments/international-covenant-economic-social-and-cultural-rights

United Nations. (1999). *Implementation of the international covenant on economic, social and cultural rights* (E/C.12/1999/10). Committee on economic, social and cultural rights (21st session). https://digitallibrary.un.org/record/407275?ln=en

World Bank. (2017, October 20). *Countries commit to strong action on human capital to drive economic growth* [Feature story]. https://www.worldbank.org/en/news/feature/2017/10/20/countries-commit-to-strong-action-on-human-capital-to-drive-economic-growth

Chapter 5
Characteristics of the Older Learner and Learning in the Later Years

5.1 The Culmination of Human Development in the Later Years

An old Hasidic proverb captures the essence of learning in the later years: For the unlearned, old age is winter; for the learned, it is the season of the harvest. Some adults achieve previously unthinkable learning achievements in later life. The Guinness World Records certified Shigemi Hirata, Japan, born on September 1, 1919, as the oldest person to receive a Bachelor of Arts degree at the age of 96 years and 200 days when he graduated from the Kyoto University of Arts and Design on March 19, 2016. It took him 11 years to complete the Ceramic Arts Program (Guinness World Records, 2023). Longevity may even affect the subjective view of age. As people grow older, they define 'old age' in terms of more years than their current age (Logan et al., 1992).

One is never too old to learn. Learning is accumulated over the lifetime – improving, correcting and updating knowledge and experience. The notion of human development is not generally associated with people in the last couple of decades of their life. But all life organisms grow and develop until they die and humans are no exception. Life is a process of development which peaks in the later years of life. Learning can support and even alter life outcomes because it helps people to understand the changing environment in which life is lived and to thrive in it. The value of learning does not change over life so long as the objectives of learning adapt to the needs in each phase of life. A prolonged life span creates urgent pressure to develop learning in later life, to ensure that the benefits of learning accrue until the end of life.

Based on the concept of senescence, old age was once considered a diagnosed disease. Healthy aging is a rebuttal. It is the means for people to be and do what they value, thereby linking personal growth, wellbeing and learning to this process of human development (World Health Organization [WHO], 2020). Three factors

S. Brink, *The Longevity Dividend*, International Perspectives on Aging 39,
https://doi.org/10.1007/978-3-031-35335-2_5

commonly associated with successful aging are good health and the absence of disease; the maintenance of cognitive and physical functioning; and active engagement in life (Fiocco & Yaffe, 2010). Learning has the potential to contribute to all three while enhancing satisfaction with life. Learning also provides spinoff effects such as building positive self-esteem, maintaining independence, building networks and increasing social engagement.

5.2 Lack of Data and Research on Learning in the Later Years

Statistical systems were designed before the phenomenon of population aging was recognized. However, statistics also predicted population aging decades before it happened, but many collections continue to sample only up to age 65 or to use '65 and over' as the last age category. For example, the OECD Survey of Adult Skills collects international data on foundational skills up to age 65 although foundational skills are known to decline with age (OECD, 2018). Variables of interest in the later years are also not collected. This makes it impossible to conduct fine-grained research on the impacts of relevant variables on disaggregated populations between 65 years and 100 or more. Women tend to dominate the older years, and they age in different ways than men. Large public programs such as public health, pensions and social service would benefit from better data. A census every 5 years remains the primary data source in many countries. When periodic surveys are conducted the samples of older persons are often too small to be statistically reliable or accurately distributed geographically. When the later years are studied, the focus is often on diseases and disabilities rather than painting the overall picture of aging, which is necessary for determining lifelong learning choices.

5.3 Participation in Learning in the Later Years

Since learning is a natural activity of life, some learning does continue in the later years. Often organized learning activities are not customized for this older cohort. There is not much data on the content of such learning or the place of its provision.

5.3.1 Learning Activities in Later Years

What little research is available indicates that people in later life do not participate in formal learning as they did at earlier ages and that they rely largely on informal learning. Formal learning activities tend to decline in later years compared to working years.

Table 5.1 Participation in learning by age and gender

	Age			
Sample	18–24	25–49	50–74	75 and older
Total sample	64%	44%	30%	13%
Men	66%	41%	29%	12%
Women	62%	46%	30%	13%
Weighted base	533	2146	1686	464

Reproduced from Learning through life: Inquiry into the future for lifelong learning by Schuller and Watson (2009) with permission from National Learning and Work Institute

The Inquiry into the Future of Lifelong Learning in the United Kingdom found a significant decline in participation in learning after age 75 (Schuller & Watson, 2009). The results are summarized in Table 5.1, where wide variation in participation underlies the average percentages.

The General Social Survey in Australia exceptionally had data for people aged 65–84 as well as 85 and over and provided information on participation in the most recent 12 months in three categories: education and training, adult education and other recreation or special interest group. While participation in formal education dropped in post-retirement, participation by those 55 to 75 and 75 and over continued into the later years. It is noteworthy that participation of 13.2% in the 75–84 age cohort was higher than the average 12.9% across all age groups (Golding et al., 2009).

Sweden has a long tradition of adult learning through 'folk schools' and learning circles. Among people with similar education, people older than 75 years were found to engage in learning as much as those 65–75 years old (Bjursell et al., 2017). It was difficult, however, for this age cohort to participate in formal learning.

In the United States, nearly 300,000 students aged 55 and older were enrolled in higher education and 21.5% of the population aged 70 years and older were enrolled in some form of lifelong learning or adult education in 2014 (Whitbourne & Montepare, 2017). Older people faced structural barriers, such as a lack of student aid and funding programs, as well as support services, such as tech support for computer aided or on-line learning (DiSilvestro, 2013).

5.3.2 *Some Informal Learning Occurs in Later Life*

Jarvis (2004) recognized the life-enriching value of informal learning, which occurred through experiential learning and learning by participation. Compared to the difficulties of formal learning or online learning for the later years cohort, informal learning offers freedom of choice and informality in organization and delivery. Among people 75 and over, 30% reported learning on their own and 14% said they learned independently with others (McNair, 2009, 2012).

Explicit or implicit informal learning occurs during participation in leisure activities or recreation with community-based groups. This can result in confidence arising from recognition of the participants' experience and strategies for tackling similar problems (MacKean & Abbott-Chapman, 2011). The groups resemble communities of practice, where likeminded people share knowledge and skills in an enjoyable way (Wenger et al., 2002). Community activities generate social capital and serve as sources of informal and incidental learning for participants (de Carteret, 2008).

Travel experiences and exposure to the culture of other countries is not always recognized as a learning venture by the voyager. However, there is a well-established market for the older traveler, who has both the time and the means. For instance, in New Zealand the median age of cruise passengers was 65 years in 2017 (65 years was the midpoint of the age frequency distribution) (Stats NZ, 2020). Some travel experiences are specialized tours to places of interest to older persons, with special lectures and a convenient pace.

5.4 The Late-life Learner

Though learners of any age share characteristics with other age cohorts, each age cohort also has special characteristics and needs. The capacity to learn among late-life learners may vary due to sensory issues or slower uptake, but motivation is key. How much they practice lifelong learning will depend on whether they see this time of life as an extraordinary opportunity to learn or if they disengage, believing that they cannot learn or doubting the value of learning for their future.

5.4.1 Cognitive Capacity and Development in Later Life

Ideas resulting from early brain research persist, suggesting that cognitive capacity declines as aging affects brain functions. The belief that the brain develops at a rapid pace in early childhood, that mental prowess peaks in young adulthood and cognitive abilities start to slowly decline after middle age is untrue. Since the Nobel prize was awarded in 2000 for the discovery of the physiological basis of memory storage in neurons in the brain, there is evidence that the brain is a highly dynamic and constantly reorganizing system throughout life. More discoveries continue to be revealed.

The Brain Changes During the Life Span

Just like the rest of the body, the brain changes continuously throughout life as an individual develops. Some changes appear negative and others more positive as the brain is a resilient organ.

Early research evidence, since replicated, showed that the volume of the brain declines by about 5% per decade after age 40 and perhaps at a faster rate after age 70. The neuronal volume may decline but not necessarily the number of neurons (Peters, 2006). Neurogenesis is the generation of new brain cells and connections between neurons. Neural stem cells produce neural cells of any type as required depending on brain stimulation. Neuroplasticity is the lifelong capacity of the human brain to change by rewiring itself. There is growing evidence that neuroplasticity or structural remodeling of the brain continues until death, allowing individuals to manage change, face new challenges and adapt to life experiences throughout life. Neuroplasticity and neurogenesis work together for brain health.

Slower processing may also be further complicated due to changes in the way sensory input is received by the brain in later life. Sensory functions such as sight and hearing may not be as acute as in the younger years (Table 5.2). However, the brain develops adaptive strategies. Human sensory systems receive vastly more information per second than the normal brain can process. The eyes receive ten million bits of information per second, but the brain can process only about 50 bits per second (Markowsky, 2023). Evolution has solved this discrepancy by ensuring that the approximately 100 billion interconnected brain cells compress and chunk the input. In order to execute billions of operations per second, some actions such as walking are automatic which allows multiprocessing.

Late-life learners may have lower capacity than the human average, which can affect both reception, chunking and processing and thus slowing learning. Information overload is when there is so much information at one time that the individual is no longer able to use the information, effectively reducing learning efficiency. Exposure to information does not necessarily mean learning. So, the presentation of information has to be paced for learning in later life.

Table 5.2 Prevalence of mild hearing and vision loss among Canadians aged 60–85, 2016

Sensory loss	Age	Men (%)	Women (%)
Mild hearing loss			
	60–64	16.2	10.2
	65–69	27.8	16.7
	70–74	38.3	29.2
	75–79	57.1	46.4
	80–85	75.9	64.8
Mild vision loss			
	60–64	23.9	27.9
	65–69	32.3	33.7
	70–74	40.9	44.3
	75–79	45.5	51.5
	80–85	56.9	58.7

Reproduced from The prevalence of hearing, vision, and dual sensory loss in older Canadians: An analysis of data from the Canadian Longitudinal Study on Aging by Mick et al. (2021) with permission from Cambridge University Press

Brain Function in Later Life

While some cognitivefunctions weaken with age, others improve through brain adaption. Life experiences and exposure to learning shape the brain across the whole life span. Depending on the life trajectory, the factors that affect cognitive function in life will be specific to an individual and the stage of life. This results in individual variations in rates of change, with some people performing well in advanced years and others less so. Though the health of neurons and their connectivity are necessary for brain function, indirect factors also have an impact.

Older adults have accumulated a lifetime of knowledge and experiences, which they apply with varying skill to real life challenges (Schaie, 1996). Further research is needed to fully understand individual variations in brain function, but there are some hypotheses. Neuronal changes may themselves vary in extent and importance between individuals. Some individuals may be more adaptive in relying on behavioral and social factors, taking greater advantage of the opportunities and environment to promote growth and function of their cognitive functions.

Of the four memory functions, episodic and semantic memory may start to decline as early as age twenty, while procedural and working memory are less affected (Peters, 2006). Nevertheless, the different cognitive functions have different life courses (Schaie, 1996). In general, as people age, they improve at detecting relationships between diverse bits of information and constructing the big picture and the wider implications of specific issues. While older persons may do less abstract thinking, formation of new concepts and verbal and numeric reasoning, they compensate by retaining their skills that are well practiced and almost automatic. Neurobiological evidence suggests that the brains of older people are better able to allocate its mental resources (Goldberg, 2006). Older brains use shared patterns in the stock of memories and experiences to structure them into competencies and expertise on which they can draw when needed. Experience enables the use of these structured competencies and expertise to solve problems efficiently.

The brain of an older person can be more efficient, choosing the path that consumes the least energy to optimize functioning in order to sort out viable options for making decisions or solving problems (Martins et al., 2012). In the teenage and young adult years, the brain develops many partitioned networks with high inner connectivity for the specialized processing necessary for the knowledge and skills learned at that stage. When people reach their forties, the brain has fewer specialized connections between separate networks but grows more connected globally across networks. When people are in their eighties, the brain is less regionally specialized but integrated and interconnected. There is neurobiological evidence that with growing age both brain hemispheres are used simultaneously. These changes affect cognition. Older adults tend to have rich vocabularies and greater understanding of the meaning of words (Hoffman, 2018). They may also increase vocabulary and general knowledge as they grow older.

Normal aging does not include major deterioration in cognitive capacity though there are changes in the brain. This was demonstrated through the Seattle Longitudinal Study, which tracked the cognitive abilities of thousands of people aged 50 and over. There was no uniform pattern of changes across cognitive abilities due to increasing age. In some cases, these older adults performed better on tests of verbal abilities, spatial reasoning, math and abstract reasoning than they did when they were younger! Though fluid cognitive abilities start to decline earlier, their crystallized abilities were affected only in the late seventies. Even at age 81, less than half of individuals in the sample had an observable decline in cognitive capacity over the 7 years of the study (Schaie, 1984). Disuse was a factor in any decline among community dwelling older people. Furthermore, such losses were reversible. With cognitive training approximately two-thirds of those that had losses showed significant improvement. About 40% of older people that declined over 14 years returned to their original levels (Schaie & Willis, 2010). In fact, the inability to learn new information may be an early indication of cognitive disease in an aging person. These facts suggests that lifelong learning can make a difference in healthy brain function.

Learning Makes the Difference Between Growing Old and Living Long

Brain imaging has shown that learning and mental activity were not only outcomes of brain function but also that learning can shape neural connections, synapses and brain structure (Centre for Educational Research and Analysis, 2007; OECD, 2002). While normal activities and familiar routines can stimulate existing brain cells, it is the learning of new knowledge, skills and experiences that creates new connections between neurons and develops greater mental growth and flexibility. In fact, learning is important for brain health (Milstein, 2022). Simultaneously learning multiple skills is feasible for healthy older adults (Leanos et al., 2020). There are nevertheless some factors that serve as barriers to learning.

Literacy and Numeracy Decline with Age

Controlling for cohort effects, the rate of literacy decline with age is quite pronounced in selected OECD countries. In Canada, the decline is even more pronounced with age at lower percentiles of literacy proficiency (Barrett & Riddell, 2019). Higher rates of literacy and numeracy are likely to moderate cognitive aging.

The foundational skills of literacy and numeracy are strongly correlated with lifelong learning. These foundational skills are learned in early education. If they are poorly acquired at that time, the deficiency contributes to growing inequalities over the lifetime with serious consequences for major outcomes, such as work, earnings, health and life expectancy. In a life-course perspective, educational inequalities accumulate, and because they affect all future learning they have an effect on the acquisition of human capital over the life course. Lower capacity to learn results in reduced human capital, which in turn affects social, economic and wellbeing outcomes in later years of life. Due to such inequities, the people who would benefit the most from lifelong learning are unable to benefit from it. As the individual's human capital stock protects against unexpected lifetime challenges, adverse events and external shocks, it is worthwhile to improve or at least maintain literacy and numeracy even in older ages.

Stereotype Threat

Anxiety may result from the risk of confirming an undesirable stereotype (Steele & Aronson, 1995). The stereotype can relate to aging, such as older people cannot learn. Such stereotype threats have been blamed for dispositional barriers that cause negative self-perception and low expectations that cause fewer older learners to participate in learning activities. Further, this could result in negative perception of one's aging, leading to underperformance and withdrawal from society. It is important to frame aging as part of human development and as a valid and meaningful part of life. If there were positive perceptions of the learning of older people, they could experience a 'stereotype boost' (Shih et al., 2012) when they would learn better than expected.

5.4.2 Learner Characteristics

The range of characteristics related to varying age and health are the most obvious identifiers of learners in later life. However, these learners have a wider life experience, too. They have lived longer and are healthier and more active than previous generations. While they have some shared experiences, these cohorts are the most diverse and varied with regard to individual life experiences over sixty or more years of life, compared to learners of other age groups. Table 5.3 presents a selection of relevant characteristics.

These characteristics should not mask the positive characteristics of older learners, such as maturity, self-confidence, purposefulness, open-mindedness, experience and receptiveness to change. Older learners share some characteristics with other learners such as curiosity, reflectiveness and readiness to investigate new ideas. They may also have high expectations that their effort to learn will not be a waste of their time and money and that what they learn can be applied immediately. Their learning orientation tends to be challenge-based or need- and problem-driven.

For those who indulge, learning can offer adventure, challenging exploration and satisfaction from success. It feeds one's curiosity, need for stimulation, thirst for novelty and search for new experiences. These side benefits of the learning journey are the same regardless of age and may motivate lifelong learners.

Table 5.3 Learner characteristics relevant to learning in later life

Learner characteristics relevant to learning in later life			
Health	Education and skills	Income and work	Life experiences
Healthier but may have manageable chronic conditions Levels of foundational skills and cognitive ability vary among individuals Exercise more and are more active but may have reduced physical strength Could still drive and travel but not all are able to May use mobility aids Diminished ability to regulate body temperature resulting in high use of energy for heating indoor spaces Majority live independently but some live in collective settings with care May be lonely or have poor mental health	More educated than previous generations with complex transitions and learning pathways Could have gained from workplace training May not have taken a formal course since retirement Literacy and numeracy skills could decline Varied demand for learning, often self-managed and directed Interested in national and global context Varied levels of digital proficiency and access May have lower expertise on financial instruments and may have been victims of scams	Generally, financially independent and if not, supported by public programs Saving for retirement for up to a time horizon of 100 years and a third of life Could have fixed retirement incomes More varied work histories for both men and women Many have held professional and responsible jobs Many provide volunteer service in charitable, cultural or sports sector	May have a spouse, children and grandchildren May have experienced bereavement and widowhood Could have reduced social networks due to deaths of contacts and reduced opportunities for interaction Greater variation in interests and expectations for later years Have established values, beliefs and opinions

Author's elaboration, 2023

5.5 Learning Needs in the Later Years

Learning can offer a window into a world that, while reaching into the past, outfits a person with competencies to thrive in the present and build a desirable future. This requires understanding how personal learning needs for day-to-day living and for anticipated future needs can be met by developing competencies.

A competency is a proven or demonstrated individual capacity to use knowledge and skills in order to meet routine, changing or new situations in life (UNESCO, n.d.). A competency bundles knowledge, skills and attitudes together so they can ensure good performance at the right time and for the proper purpose. Knowledge is the required information, including theories, facts and successful solutions, and the ability to apply this information appropriately to different situations. Skills are the trained ability to act based on practice and to choose and perform the right technique at the right time. It is usually developed through training and practice. Attitudes are values expressed through what is thought and felt. Competencies composed of these elements are observable and transferable (UNESCO, n.d.).

In the later years, an individual is expected to manage their own learning. The process includes scanning the time and context of their life, evaluating needs and interests, researching the options that could satisfy the needs, choosing an option for the time and type of learning, engaging in learning and integrating learning to add to personal competencies. The choice from an array of possibilities is based more on the desired competency rather than on age. The learner may have their own preferences and their developed patterns of learning from past experience. There are many paths to learning and none of them are wrong so long as they work for the individual learner.

5.5.1 Learning Needs Derive from the Demands of Later Life

The expected multiple societal roles expected in later life can be grouped into four broad goals (Brink, 2021).

Life management. Learning to understand aging in relation to the specific situation of an individual who, to succeed in life, adapts at a pace responsive to changes in the living context.

Personal development. To lead a life of purpose by directing personal growth, first by understanding the natural, economic, social and political world in which a person seeks to succeed and second by developing one's interests, talents and natural abilities to thrive in that context.

Societal contributions. To learn to maximize knowledge and abilities to contribute to family, community and society commensurate with personal capacity.

Legacy for the future. To transmit experience, ideas and infrastructure for future generations.

Every individual may choose their own program of learning to meet these goals, depending on the opportunities and the available time, energy and capability for learning. There are no rigid expectations of how the goals should be met, but it is clear that learning and meeting the goals result in making later life more successful and satisfying.

Examples of specific competencies related to the societal roles of a well-rounded person in later years under the four goals of later life are shown in Tables 5.4a, 5.4b, 5.4c and 5.4d. They are noted alongside generic competencies. Other age groups would be interested in gaining generic competencies, but the specific competencies of later years would not likely be of the same priority for them as for people in their later years. If this was nonetheless the case, learning options can be offered to the

Table 5.4a Competencies related to the later life goal of life management

Goal: Life management		
Role of person in later life in society	Generic competencies (examples)	Specific competencies (examples)
Manage personal health and wellbeing	Importance of healthy living activities such as diet, exercise Maintaining a diverse social network	Understanding age related health conditions and their management through self-care, including therapeutic diets, medications and fall avoidance, mental health Maintaining an active and diverse social network Types of exercise possible given health status (e.g., chair yoga, Aqua Fit) Information on sensory loss and its mitigation Prevention and quick diagnosis of major illnesses such as heart attacks and strokes Ability to make informed decisions about palliative care and assisted death
Prudent financial management	Personal finance – budget, loans and taxes Socially responsible investing	Budgets, loans, taxes applicable to retired status; pension management; investment instruments; divestment; prepaid funerals and burials; safe use of banking services for seniors; protection against scams and fraud
Wise consumer	Energy saving purchases – car, refrigerator, home insulation Circular economy (reduce, reuse, recycle)	Informed decision when and where to downsize or to move to collective housing; On-line purchasing of aging related products
Legal	Purchase or sale of property	Purchase or sale of property; wills and estate planning, bequests, major donations

Author's elaboration, 2023

public of any age for generic competencies while targeting older people in their later years for specific competencies without excluding others.

The older person has multiple competing demands clamouring for more information to support the decisions and actions in later life. The priorities chosen for learning are deeply personal.

5.6 Learning Processes and Adaptations in Later Years

Lifelong learning may not be a specific goal for all older people. The idea of lifelong learning came to be used only in the 1960s. The bundle of competencies around learning-to-learn was not part of the curriculum for those who finished secondary school before then. They would not have been taught to make lifelong learning a daily activity, like exercise. Thus, their learning processes and preferences are determined by their own personal learning trajectory.

Table 5.4b Competencies related to the later life goal of personal development

Goal: Personal development		
Role of person in later life in society	Generic competencies (examples)	Specific competencies (examples)
Information and communication to understand the life-world context	Evaluate the accuracy, reliability and credibility of information in order to use or share valid, appropriate information; media literacy	Informed, political and scientific advances related to health and aging; evaluate the accuracy, reliability and credibility of information related to later years in order to use or share valid appropriate information; media literacy Best individual fit of available public aging or older person programs
Personal interests	Updating marketable skills	Updating skills; improve digital competence; passion projects such as memoir writing, genealogy or painting; learning a second language
Recreation and culture	Theatre, art museums, libraries	Theatre, art museums, libraries, particularly with special programs and performances/ products for older people; aging oriented library services including mobile services; choices that increase social activity such as choirs, book clubs and learning circles; learning through travel (e.g., Roads scholars)

Author's elaboration, 2023

Table 5.4c Competencies related to the later life goal of societal contributions

Goal: Societal contributions		
Role of person in later life in society	Generic competencies (examples)	Specific competencies (examples)
Care giving	Caring roles in the family	Caring for a spouse with special needs; seeking complementary professional and social services care (e.g., respite care)
Grand parenting	Intergenerational relationships	Care and nurturing for mutual benefit of child and grandparent
Work	Updating work related knowledge and skills	Knowledge and skills that can be used for current occupation (full or part-time or consulting) or for second (encore) career
Volunteering	Knowledge and skills that support volunteering	Skills in demand in the community or on-line such as editing, teaching English or other as second language

Author's elaboration, 2023

5.6.1 Learning-to-Learn in Later Life

Learning-to-learn consists of beliefs, behaviours, emotions and strategies that facilitate the acquisition of knowledge and skills to advance the understanding of the world and life contexts. It facilitates storage and retrieval of knowledge for application to appropriate situations, to improve results or to apply solutions to new

Table 5.4d Competencies related to the later life goal of legacy for the future

Goal: Legacy for the future		
Role of person in later life in society	Generic competencies (examples)	Specific competencies (examples)
Next generation	Record family life	Provide a family history, photographic record, family artifacts, genealogy to younger generations
Carriers of culture and tradition	Build family traditions	Transmit family traditions, traditional language, music and cuisine to the larger family
Citizenship responsibilities	Knowledge about current issues such as climate change and solutions for the future in order to make good voting choices Sustainable development	Knowledge about current issues such as climate change and solutions for the future in order to make good voting choices; social innovations and investment; sharing memories of collective history
World citizen	World view Transmitting importance of world citizenship to children	National and international philanthropy; activism for collective wellbeing and survival of the species

Author's elaboration, 2023

contexts (Weinstein et al., 2010). Metacognition, or thinking about and understanding one's own learning, is an important personal skill.

Older people take responsibility for their own learning-to-learn when they need to, depending on what they find meaningful for successful living, and thereby add to their store of knowledge (Illeris, 2006). Learning may occur in different times in life due to interaction with different actors, varying venues and ways of learning. The process of lifelong learning itself thus has a learning component. To benefit from lifelong learning, people need to learn how to learn even in later life.

Learning-to-learn is also facilitated by the foundational skills for learning. These are the skills, such as literacy, numeracy and digital skills, that facilitate the process of learning and strongly affect learning performance. Literacy and numeracy are known to decline with age if not maintained, and digital skills are new and evolving. All these skills need to be learned and maintained through continuous effort.

Learning-to-learn may also require learning in new ways. People in later life may not have taken on-line courses before. Though they may have learned to use digital devices, learning at a distance or in a digital course that requires asynchronous learning may be a new experience.

5.6.2 Relearning and Updating

Cognitive disuse may limit the cognitive performance of people in later life. Depending on their learning activities in earlier years, people in their later years may have forgotten some of what they had previously learned. If they have not learned new material, their stock of knowledge may be out of date. These changes could result in the loss of human capital and a decline in its relevance for meeting current needs. People may need to refresh their knowledge and to learn some totally new content if new knowledge builds on new concepts.

5.6.3 Design of Later Learning for Knowledge Acquisition, Retention and Application

Educational gerontology is the study of changes in the learning processes caused by old age. Other factors also change the learning processes. The field of learning in later life is in its nascency, but some good practices can be described. There is tremendous diversity in the later life age group because it includes three or more cohorts of a decade each. This has two consequences for the provision of learning. First, learning design or provision cannot be standardized. Age-based curricula are not realistic. The challenge is the greatest where there are learners of multiple age cohorts. Personalization and customization are important. Second, the diversity of needs, human capital and learning experience in later life means that learners expect choice among a variety of options in both content and provision. Designing for the extreme or the average are poor solutions for this large and growing age group.

5.6.4 The Learning Flowline Is Generic But May Be Customized by the Later Life Learner

The three recognized learning phases apply regardless of age and stage of life. Each learner orchestrates his or her cognitive resources and learning-to-learn skills to achieve the selected learning goal. Issues with any one phase or more can result in partial, poor or no learning at all. Even if information is understood, if it is not integrated it cannot be recalled for later use.

The Learning Moment and the Consequent Readiness to Learn

The need for knowledge and skills creates the demand for learning. When the timing is right, there is peak personal engagement in the learning moment. During this phase, an older learner evaluates his or her own human capital in relation to the life context, undertakes environmental scanning, priorizes learning needs, examines opportunities, selects the best option and organizes access for the learning required.

The Active Learning Phase

The older learner engages in learning and maximizes its effectiveness by using learning skills to evaluate its validity, to practice and test the new information and to gauge when and how it can be used. Mere exposure to materials to be learned is insufficient without building on previous personal learning and understanding the new knowledge enough to apply it appropriately in future situations.

Integration into Human Capital and Conversion into Competence

In this phase the older learner recognizes the value of what was learned and creates meaning. New knowledge is reinforced, consolidated and assimilated. This means integrating it with prior knowledge and experience and storing it in easily retrievable memory for use when required. The process helps to determine the general and specific applications for transference to other times and contexts.

5.6.5 Choice of Opportunities for Learning in Later Years

The lack of choice in content, type and length of course or program and mode of delivery is a key issue for older learners. It arises due to several reasons.

Lack of Standardized Design Creates Complexity

Equity requires that all late-life learners have access to the learning they need. However, after initial education, there is no organized standardized system working to move people through the pipeline to build human capital throughout life in a homogenous and consistent way. Rather, society benefits from the diversity in the potential of its members and their specialized and individual knowledge and skills. Among older people, dynamic interactions between biological, psychological, and social contexts reciprocally affect the way learning occurs (Smith & Thelen, 1994). Thus, in the later years, there is a great range of needs in a diverse population, and not all people will require the same learning at the same time in their lives. The ways in which learning occurs in later life could therefore be distinguished from that of other ages because people's starting human capital and their learning needs are both individual. They make self-directed learning decisions to build their own independent learning trajectories (Cross, 1981). By doing so, they expect transformative learning that could change the way they think about themselves and the world in which they live (Mezirow, 2000).

Public Listings of Available Learning Offerings for Later life Are Difficult to Find

Environmental scanning and selecting learning options from available choices may be complex, since there are no established places where learning opportunities for later life are consolidated nor any catalogues listing descriptions. It takes work to put together a personalized package of learning based on needs (see Tables 5.4a, 5.4b, 5.4c and 5.4d). Options may not be available in the desired order, with the preferred content or delivered by the appropriate professionals such as lawyers. Providers such as Universities of the Third Age offer choices, but not all high priority learning options may be offered. Options may not be well distributed geographically. Not all learners wish to learn remotely. Course credits are rare.

Accessibility

Accessibility is a combination of the provision of the right mix of content, the amount of time and effort needed to take advantage of the offering, the fees and the cost for travel or digital access. Accessibility is more complicated for older learners because it depends on the geographical location, which affects the learning environment and the design and delivery of learning.

Accessible Learning Locations

The ideal is to have easily accessible learning options in places where older people are concentrated. Nursing homes and retirement communities provide courses and activities, but they tend to focus on leisure and recreation. The dispersal of older people in the community makes access difficult, particularly because many live alone in their family home and some no longer drive. For example, in 2021 in Canada, 29% of those aged 75–84 years and 42% of those 85 and over lived in a one-person household (Statistics Canada, 2022). Ideally, any face-to-face learning options should be in the neighbourhood, like a community centre. It helps if locations can be reached by public transport. Innovative solutions have been used to take learning to older people rather than to move older people to learning. This can involve mobile options such as a suitably equipped bus or truck and pop-up options in libraries and parks.

Barrier-Free Learning Venues

Accessibility implies that the learning venues and the learning provided can be used comfortably by mobility or sensory impaired people and people in later life. The locations should be accessed on the ground floor or by elevators, spacious enough for wheel chairs and walkers, well heated (in cold climates), lit and ventilated and with accessible toilet facilities nearby.

5.6.6 Provision and Delivery Customized for Learners in Their Later Years

Each period of the lifespan has its own needs and challenges, which requires adaptive strategies. Older learners require adaptive customization of learning to ensure greater outreach and better outcomes for late-life learners.

Timing and Flexible Scheduling

Some choice in time of the offering and flexibility in organization of learning options can increase participation. Participating in evening or night courses may be difficult for some.

Content, Design and Delivery

Structure

It is important to structure learning in an easy-to-understand progression that can be understood regardless of age, prior knowledge or life experience. Repetition, assessment of comprehension and reinforcement to ensure learning are essential elements. Examples, exercises and practical sessions must be appropriate to later life. Successful learning involves older people being able to relate the learning to their unique knowledge base and link it to their life experience.

Duration

Self-learning is often intermittent and focused on a selected topic. Many learning themes and topics, such as preparation of wills, lend themselves to courses of short duration. However, those that are linked to lifestyle, like yoga, may be periodic over time. Those that require practice and training, such as playing bridge or genealogy, may be longer term. Some may prefer the option of learning at their own pace rather than on a fixed schedule, working on course segments on demand. As many older people are results oriented, they appreciate certification. The granting of micro-credentials related to a specific skill holds promise.

Class Size and Composition

Class size and composition matter for the older age group. Large formal classes can provide economies of scale, but they may be less than ideal for people in their later years. Discussion can be hard to manage in a large group. Sessions of smaller groups, offered more frequently, may be a better solution. Intergenerational composition is possible, but there can be considerable cohort diversity among older people even in small groups.

Digital Learning

Technology is now completely integrated into contemporary life for work, recreation, consumption, services and relating to government. Digital learning can provide learners with competencies while preparing them to incorporate technology into daily life. Digital skills facilitate participation in modern life and have the added benefit of keeping pace with fast-evolving technology.

Learning providers are attracted to digital learning, because they can build an inventory of recorded courses by experts. These can be provided on demand, offering self-managed flexibility to learners. The use of digital devices and internet in today's oldest cohort of later learners is less common than in the youngest cohort but will increase among future later learners. In Canada in 2020, 92% of the population used the internet. The percentage in the 65 to 74 age group was quite close at 86% and considerably higher than the 62% in 75 and over age group (Statistics Canada, 2021). A large share of people in the older age group will thus in a few years have some digital skills. Digitally supported learning and on-line learning can potentially grow in popularity as more older people have digital skills. But technological advances are rapid, so digital skills cannot be static. The acquisition and updating of digital skills may become a priority for all ages, including in later life.

On-line learning could be a solution for older people who are not mobile, but it is not an ideal fit because of the rapid technological changes. When on-line learning is possible, it has multiple advantages. Pre-course material can ensure that the learner has the appropriate background, and course material can be stored and reviewed whenever necessary. Flexibility of personal scheduling is offered, so learners can log-on at convenient times, from any location using different devices. Self-pacing is a plus. Learners can delay response to a time when they are prepared for interaction. Information can be presented in multiple ways, with a choice of practice exercises and additional materials.

A downside of digital learning is that learning is predicated on the learner having sufficient digital skills. Older learners may be disadvantaged by poor connectivity and unstable or expensive wifi connections. Though digital learning has been promoted for learners who are in wheel chairs or in bed, the long screen time required may be an obstacle. Only limited interaction with other students and instructors can be isolating, especially for those living alone.

5.6.7 *Late-life Pedagogy and Learning Resources*

The process of learning by older adults may be different compared to their earlier life stages. Late-life pedagogy or geragogy grew from the recognition that older learners have characteristic needs and are sufficiently different from learners of other ages to necessitate a distinct educational theoretical framework. Older learners can be participants in defining the learning curriculum and in ensuring that delivery is sensitive to their sensory and learning needs. Older learners demand that outcomes be practical and relevant to their lives in later years and societal demands. The learning process needs to draw on their experiences and rely on discussion among learners to ensure future relevance (Findsen & Formosa, 2011). The learning of older adults nonetheless remains a relatively under-researched, yet highly significant, area of educational enquiry (Formosa, 2002). Although late-life pedagogy is a growing field, there is no national certification in most countries. Demand for such knowledge and skills is likely to grow as populations age.

Learning resources for topics that are relevant for older learners are being developed. The obvious requirements are that the content be relevant to late-life learners and that the information is presented specifically for use by older adults. For instance, examples need to be meaningful for that audience and material would use large print.

Subject Expertise and Teaching Experience

Experience in working with older learners is valuable for teacher led programs for late-life learners. Unlike in a discipline, say statistics, where one single professor can teach several courses over months, several experts may be employed for shorter periods. The person leading on investment instruments would be different from the person with knowledge about powers of attorney, for example. Experience with the variety of methods they can use to ensure effective learning by older learners is a useful complement. Those who lead the learning must be able to use real life examples relevant to later life (Knowles, 1980), which they may not have experienced. However, they can draw on the real life experiences of participants.

Collaborative Learning

Collaborative learning among co-learners may be valued more among late-life learners than younger learners. Older people are open to learning through discussion, to comparing experiences, to examining wider perspectives and to sharing their expertise. Case studies, where a group may collaboratively figure out solutions can be useful. Collaboration can be used to review and validate learning from personal experiences through questions that resolve alternative perspectives (Taylor,

1998). Explaining to others the ideas learned helps to consolidate learning and to create meaning from various viewpoints.

Customization for Late-life Learners

Personalization and presentation from a well-established starting point allow learners to self-assess their prior learning. Multiple teaching and learning strategies with reiteration and repetition can help those who prefer an alternate method of learning or a slower pace. Where possible, self-pacing may be preferred. Immediate feedback related to the learning objective helps both the teacher and the late-life learner to determine how to improve comprehension of the subject matter (Taylor, 1998).

Adjustments for Diverse Sensory and Cognitive Capacities

Because of the range of sensory and cognitive capacities, stamina and concentration among late-life learners, it is wise to check periodically that presentations and resource materials are comfortable for them to use. Adaptations may be made to font size in print or screen. The sound quality and volume should be adjusted when visual aids or videos are used. Speed of subtitles and scrolling may need to be slowed (Knowles, 1980; Knowles and Associates, 1984).

5.7 General Learning Approaches for Late-life Learners

While each of the following learning approaches is in wide use for the general public, they are not equally effective for learners in later life. Prior experience and preferences of late-life learners can play a role in their effectiveness. These approaches are offered by a wide variety of providers already, and they may adapt them to meet the needs of late-life learners.

5.7.1 Self-Directed Independent Learning

Children, particularly young children, learn independently when engaged in play, exploration and experimentation. The skills required for learner autonomy and learning-to-learn are honed from childhood as people develop over their life course. Among late-life learners, independent learning includes many skills. They include the ability to identify their knowledge needs, to jettison their outdated ways of thinking, to seek the best match for the learning goals they set, to rely on appropriate resources using logic and inference to contextualize information, to evaluate the information for relevance, bias and truth, to marshal the effort and time required in a self-disciplined way and to self-evaluate their own learning critically and with maturity.

As early as the 1970s, it was believed that the bulk of adult learning was self-directed. Research confirmed this. Approximately 70% of adult learning is self-directed and about 90% of all adults engage in at least one self-directed project a year (Cross, 1981; Tough, 1971). Independent self-directed learning in later life can be with or without a teacher or leader who supports the learning process.

Independent or autonomous learning among older adults has been described as being 'life centered' and pragmatic because they undertake learning to satisfy their personal needs and interests (Lindeman, 1961). They are able to take charge of their personal learning and are described as self-activated and active agents in their own learning (Rathbone, 1971). The attractions are obvious, as one can learn in one's own time, own space and own pace by setting personal learning goals, designing the learning experience and assessing one's own learning. Late-life learners find such control conducive to their learning. They establish their expectations of anticipated results. They seek out the opportunities to practice new skills and appreciate the immediate feedback on their successful application of the new knowledge to an appropriate condition (Knowles, 1975). Deep learning provides the confidence that the learned knowledge has been integrated and can be retrieved and applied to unfamiliar situations and real-life scenarios when required.

5.7.2 Learning from Professionals, Experts or Specialists

Learning in later life can occur in a classroom, in groups or as private tutoring with a professional, expert or specialist. The late-life learner makes a choice of the institution, course or teacher to be confident about the authenticity of the knowledge that will be presented. Specialists are known for their skills and will be able to teach by demonstrating techniques, explain use and standards of quality, provide feedback or correction during practice and guide the mastering of a new skill (a new language, for example). The step of evaluating and validating new knowledge may thus be skipped because of confidence in the source.

Most older people have been away from formal learning for decades, and some may still be haunted by negative school experiences (Rubenson, 2011). But the need and motivation suffice for them to formulate their expectations for the learning they want to acquire. Those in the teaching role may rely on personalized approaches to present new real time knowledge and skills, while managing the process of learning and building on the existing human capital of these learners. Because of the need for personal relevance, learners may wish to set their own learning outcomes based on individual needs and assessment of their resources or capacities. They may also wish to determine the pace and pathways so that instruction can be individualized. Empowering older learners to learn autonomously requires the teacher to facilitate learning and to encourage reflection and integration of the new knowledge. Jarvis (2004) recommended that older learners be offered an array of choices, such as relying on self-knowledge to determine need, choosing to study attractive parts of a course, working at their own speed and using a preferred learning style.

5.7.3 *Teaching Based on Inquiry*

Inquiry-based teaching methods rely on using questions about an issue from different perspectives, working out potential answers and evaluating them.

Didactic Teaching

This method is based on the use of questions followed by evaluation of a range of responses for the best answer. It facilitates learning by causing learners to define the characteristics of the issue or problem, to use and question their own store of knowledge, in order to perfect the fit of their explanation by trying different responses, and to clearly explain to others the best solution and its utility (Jarvis, 2004).

Socratic Method

Late-life learners generally wish to be engaged in the learning process. The classic Socratic method is designed to make learners create their own meaning of what they learn rather than reproduce knowledge. It requires the teacher to make learners consider a logical sequence of questions, to make learners respond to each in turn by requiring them to crystalize the knowledge that they have and to add information to this base. It is an effective method for late-life learners because it utilizes a means to combine their accumulated human capital with what they have learned from life experience (Jarvis, 2004).

5.7.4 *Experiential Learning*

Late-life learners are encouraged to take responsibility for their own learning while applying their existing and new knowledge to real life issues. Learners evaluate their learning needs and processes by appropriate use of available resources, integrating new learning and applying new knowledge appropriately to new problems (Tight, 2003). These methods encourage learners to try out solutions, while making practical use of their knowledge and applying it in a way that knowledge would be used in a real life context (Goddu, 2012). Experiential techniques, such as discussion, simulation, case method and problem solving, tap into the experiences of the learner, thereby engaging adult learners (Caminotti & Gray, 2012).

Problem Based Learning

Learning can be based on real problems faced by a community, a case study of a problem that had occurred in the recent past, or a current problem of a learner. Because learning is both active and self-directed, the instructor serves as facilitator, and the students take the lead in developing the solutions. The process helps learners to evaluate their own knowledge and experience while collaborating and experimenting with real issues (Karge et al., 2011). Problem based learning makes difficult problems manageable by breaking up the process into problem identification, exploration of options and testing solutions (Tight, 2003). The method is appreciated by many older learners because they are given a real-life situation or problems and some guidelines on how to solve the problem by using existing or new information, but learning results from their own efforts.

Simulation

Simulation presents a situation where learners actively experience the resolution of an issue by proposing potential ways to address it and to evaluate and reflect on what was learned through the process. Learners build on prior knowledge by research, trial and error and weighing potential outcomes. Simulations provide learners with an environment where they can reflect on their own choices, examine the different proposals from others with similar outcomes and review what was learned (Rutherford-Hemming, 2012).

5.7.5 Narrative Learning

Late-life learners use narrative learning to form a link between lived experience and new learning content. Autobiographical life events and experiences are the start. Learners identify their value systems and test them against new concepts and ideas that arise. They learn to transcend their personal attitudes and experience to examine the larger social and cultural contexts that shaped their lives (Clark & Rossiter, 2006).

5.7.6 Collaborative Learning

Collaborative work sharpens skills through interaction with other late-life learners rather than relying solely on the instructor (Davis, 2013). Collaboration reveals how similar situations can provide different but equally valid life lessons depending on individual context.

Discussions and Seminars

Discussions work well for learners in their later years if the ground rules are clearly set to ensure everyone participates and if the purpose and expectations are clear. Discussion requires learners to find relevance in relation to their life experience and personal knowledge. They apply curiosity to their questions, critical thinking to their contributions and negotiate meaning across ideas and responses of others. Learning occurs when discussions promote higher order thinking. This arises through elaboration of ideas supported by evidence, progression of knowledge building during the give and take of discussion and reflection of key points for integration (Davis, 2013).

Group Work

The interactive environment provided when groups of learners work together facilitates group and individual learning through collaboration. Shared expertise and common enterprise lead to group affiliation for engagement as well as responsibility for group success (Scherling, 2011). Group work can also be used for a joint project, where knowledge and skills of each member is valued for the contribution to the learning of others as well as group success.

5.7.7 Peer Learning

Late-life learners shift from independent learning to interdependent learning when a two-way reciprocal mutual-learning activity is introduced through peer learning (Boud, 1988). This is a collegial process, which relies on trust and rapport with others with valuable knowledge to share. Such knowledge can arise from shared life stage experiences, life contexts, similar social issues or challenges (Beckingham & Watt, 1995). They know they can call on expert resource people if necessary, understanding that they may not be from the same age cohort or have shared similar life experiences. Learning between two or more peers working in a co-operative learning environment with achievable goals set by the group in relation to shared expected outcomes has advantages. Regardless of whether learners have extensive or little knowledge or expertise, they are equals as learners with regard to their responsibilities in the group. Learning is enhanced by free exchange of credible experiential knowledge using everyday vernacular. Peers learn more about themselves, expand their perspectives while learning from others and build meaningful connections (Boud et al., 2001).

When a learner takes on a teaching role, they work through concepts and explain their ideas in multiple ways to other peers who might learn in different ways and may share other perspectives. The learning process may evolve in unanticipated ways, which develops skills in inquiry and dialogue as well as incidental learning.

For instance, the peer learning process may help an older learner to articulate his or her own position and how it differs from the views of peers. This enables the peer group to distinguish between consensus, enrichment and dissent. In addition, peers develop skills in planning learning activities, organizing and integrating knowledge, transmitting knowledge in learning modules, giving and receiving feedback and evaluating their own learning.

5.7.8 Intergenerational and Multigenerational Learning

Formal education is often stratified by age under the assumption that the learners have achieved the same competencies and have similar learning skills. Mixed-generation settings, in contrast, are expected to encourage exchange between people who need knowledge and people who have had more exposure to such knowledge or know how to obtain it.

Intergenerational learning has been described as the exchange between any two generations, which involves the sharing of knowledge, skills and experience (Ventura-Merkel & Lidoff, 1983). Intergenerational learning can occur between people of two or more living generations or between one or more people in a living generation and one or more person in the past. Learning in the absence of the past-generation members occurs through analyzing their life histories and their legacy of contributions to recorded knowledge, skills and experience (Brink, 2021). It is a partnership based on reciprocity and mutuality with a shared learning goal. This generates additional or different benefits to those arising from single-generation learning.

Intergenerational learning results in more efficient transmission of knowledge held by every person in the setting. It has some special characteristics. The learning process is not exclusively a unidirectional flow of knowledge from one older knowledge holder to many knowledge seekers. Learning or experience is rather offered by people of any age without defining knowledge or experience in relation to any other age group. The process values the life experience and knowledge of older people that make them 'life-wise'. This implies that everyone should be a teacher, sharing their knowledge and skills at the same time as each one is also a willing learner, learning from others who have the knowledge they desire or need. Thus, in intergenerational learning the focus is shifted from age and hierarchy to the value of sharing individually held human capital regardless of the source. It severs the link between knowledge and seniority or status of individuals. It acknowledges the value of the aggregated knowledge of the group and places responsibility on each individual to share their knowledge with others while learning from them.

Intergenerational learning relies on multiple learning processes that appeal to late-life learners because each manages their own sharing and learning (Brink, 2021).

Cooperative Critical Thinking

Critical thinking is essential to fully understand the context, define the issue or situation, consider its systemic nature and develop multiple solutions approached from different angles. Because the group is composed of diverse people with different backgrounds there are no disciplinary boundaries that impede the creation of interdisciplinary solutions.

Collaborative Inquiry

Learning is always learner-centered and self-directed but builds on collective prior knowledge. Mutual interest in learning is combined with personalized inquiry associated with an individual learner's motivation, experience and need. Learners rely on questioning based on what knowledge each one has, followed by evaluating new insights based on discussion and integrating new knowledge. Questions build on each other to construct knowledge.

Updating

Discussion with others can reveal obsolescent knowledge as well as much tested wisdom. When new information or practices are introduced in society at a point in time, new knowledge and know-how can be disseminated rapidly through intergenerational learning groups since every learner can also teach another. This is especially important when knowledge and practice is too new or increasing at too rapid a rate to be absorbed into curricula in formal learning. New know-how is quickly learned through discussion and demonstration.

Co-learning

During intergenerational learning, participants are accountable for the learning of each person, while compensating for individual shortcomings and gaining from individual strengths. Learners take asymmetric roles and use one another's resources, experiences and skills to strengthen learning. Co-learning builds on the social aspects of learning: diverse people make meaning together from shared information to address new social challenges that they face in their own life context and in society. Individuals improve communication and thinking skills, while the whole group validates information within the cultural context.

Co-production

Learning is driven by demand. Co-production is a synergetic process that combines transdisciplinary knowledge, varied life and professional experiences, different levels of technical expertise and multiple work proficiencies of the learners. This mix enables the synthesizing of new knowledge and new ways of doing things through cross fertilization to address real life situations and complex contemporary societal challenges. Learners also learn how to leverage collective pools of knowledge, individual expertise, and joint investigation to generate new knowledge or know-how. The process develops individuals as knowledge brokers, bridge builders and problem solvers as they identify their own tacit and explicit knowledge stock.

5.7.9 Remote or e-Learning

Despite the prevailing perception that people in their later years are reluctant to use digital devices for learning, a large proportion own such devices. In the United States, for example, some late-life learners were interested to use their digital technology to take on-line learning or on-line tutorials (13% and 14%, respectively, of those 60–69 years and 70 and over) or to take on-line education courses for certificates or degrees (16% and 13%, respectively, of those 65–69 years and 70 and over) (AARP Research, 2021).

Remote or e-learning uses electronic media for learning through the internet, but the full value of digital learning is achieved when it is used to enhance learning. Digital learning can be synchronous, when all learners and the instructor are on line simultaneously with interactions in real time, or asynchronous, when the learner is able to control learning and the timing of a response.

Digital devices such as smart phones, tablets and laptops are widely used. Their use in learning can vary considerably. Access to reliable internet service is essential. Learning material can vary from print, graphics and videos. Some preprogrammed learning experiences can provide immediate feedback, such as the number of correct answers or an explanation. There are both advantages and disadvantages of e-learning, particularly for late-life learners (Table 5.5).

5.8 Locating Learning in Later Life in the Lifelong Learning System

It can be argued that learning in later life is the culmination of the learning trajectory of human life. It would not be surprising therefore if the learning possibilities required are rich and varied compared to the type of learning provided in earlier

Table 5.5 Remote or e-learning options and their advantages and disadvantages for late-life learners

Learning option	Advantages and disadvantages
Interactive website	Can provide information on demand. Information is written for the general public, but can have too much or too little detail
	Learners have to be cautious about accuracy
	Generally free but may require membership or registration
	Responsibility for verification and adoption rests with the user
	Risky websites are used for scamming
Webinars	Scheduled presentations on specified topics accessed through the web
	May require a fee or they can be free
	Information on availability depends on type of promotion and target audience
	International webinars may be at odd times due to the time difference. Sometimes, they are recorded and can be viewed later rather than in real time
	Timing, level of discourse and fees may not be right for late-life learners
Videos	How-to videos and presentations by well-known experts on a specific topic
	They can range from a few minutes to hour long presentations and require reliable access to the internet, good band width and preferably large enough screen for easy viewing
	Pacing, font size of text and scrolling speed can be problems for late-life learners
Text message learning	Short pieces of information sent fairly frequently to learners with smart phones on request or registration
	Has been used for example to provide key safety information every week to older workers during their break and a daily exercise for late-life learners
On-line course	Courses may be purchased or provided free and downloaded by the learner
	Length can vary depending on the subject and the provider
	Learner can learn at own pace and respond to assignments when completed
	If satisfactorily completed, some courses may provide a certificate or badge
Massive Open Online Course or MOOCs	Popular online open access, often free, courses on a variety of topics, involving universities and experts and attracting thousands of students
	Usually start at a fixed time and run for a specified number of weeks
	Content is delivered through video lectures and readings and assessments on-line. Satisfactory completion is recognized
	Some earned credits can be accepted by educational institutions or employers. Quality can vary
	There may be insufficient interaction and tech support for late-life learners
Game based or simulation	A real situation is presented to a group of learners who meet the assumptions and rules to develop and apply a potential solution to test its efficacy
	Late-life learners may not keep pace with the speed of action

Author's elaboration, 2023

years. The variation in individual lives over seven or eight decades should be respected, and suitable learning options provided to meet the diverse needs.

The learning infrastructure for the whole life must be seamless in instructing people through the life course, linking different parts of the system and offering multiple pathways for successful learning. Learning in every age in the life course should be valued, and later life should not be excluded. The system should recognize the different purposes of each learning stage and allow individuals to access them in any personalized order and at any stage of life. It should provide flexible alternatives for use by individuals of varied abilities and interests, personal life trajectories and different learning abilities or learning levels. Using the current generic system and making a few tweaks will not work for these learners in later life.

In later life, individuals should be able to learn any desired competency, using appropriate learning strategies and flexible options. Learning should build on prior knowledge and life experience. Neither age nor weaker physical or cognitive capacity should be considered limitations, since strategies exist to adapt learning accordingly. Learning options can be provided by many organizations, public, private and non-profit, but they should be available to all older people wherever they live.

Older people are very diverse in terms of their learning needs but also physical and cognitive capacities. At one end of the spectrum, people in later life can learn using the institutions, structures and options that are available for all adults and, on the other extreme, learning options may resemble individual tutoring or counselling, even at bedside. But because a majority of older people in their later years are relatively healthy, most learning options can be customized for their needs. Niche options can be developed for a minority who have specific needs. For instance, there are populations of older people in later life who live in community settings, whether retirement homes or Naturally Occurring Retirement Communities (NORC – a defined geographic area with a naturally occurring high density of residents aged 55 and over) due to aging in place. Others live in collective settings and institutions. However, many people in later life live alone and are not always mobile. Their place of residence should not limit their access to learning.

The use of existing learning offerings by late-life learners is low relative to the size of this population segment. The existing supply of potential learning options tends to attract a limited and privileged segment of older learners. Organizations such as Universities of the Third Age provide a valuable service, with a range of learning options targeting late-life learners. The majority of learners are women. However, such institutions have been criticized for being 'elitist' because the courses attract an advantaged segment of the older population. They tend to attract middle class women but do not attract men (Formosa, 2011).

Insufficiency of opportunities alone may not be the reason why older adults do not engage in learning. Given their share of the population, their demand for learning would be expected to be higher than it is. The low demand could be due to such factors as cost, inconvenience, and difficult access. Scarcity of information, poor incentives, lack of relevance, poor value of learning particular topics or a perceived lack of returns may contribute to demand being low. A better match between supply and demand could be achieved with more effective public information about the value of lifelong learning for late-life learners.

Lifelong learning is a new idea for many people in later life. Learning is voluntary and older individuals exercise agency by making choices and decisions regarding their own learning. They may be constrained, however, by cultural, social and financial factors, which affect their behaviours related to learning opportunities (Giddens, 1984). Learning may not be viewed as part of aging. Society may thus place too much emphasis on self-motivated, self-directed learning that is self-funded by late-life learners. Since learning should be considered an essential activity and a public good, the responsibility for lifelong learning is shared between the individual, society and government. Failure of the system affects society negatively over the long term.

5.9 Inequity and Learning Poverty in the Later Years

Inequity in learning can arise between stages in the life course and also within a population segment in their later years. For instance, schooling is provided to 100% of children in most countries, but provision of learning seems to decline over the life course. The number of adults engaging in training ranged from 60% in the United States to 20% in the Russian Federation (ILO, 2018). Participation declines further in old age. Only 15% of older adults engaged in learning in the United Kingdom (Schuller & Watson, 2009). Though informal learning may predominate, it cannot by itself yield the results that can be gained by a well-organized self-directed learning program. It is not systematic and some topics do not lend themselves (for example medical, legal or financial subjects) to informal learning. Though the impact of learning in later life is just as important as it is to an earlier stage of life, the majority of people do not engage in learning in later life.

The cost of inequity in learning in the later years is not well understood. Lack of learning has impacts on the individual, the population of older people and the whole of society. Individuals who engage in learning tend to experience healthy aging, higher quality of life and life satisfaction. The reasons for no learning at all can be many, but none of them can justify the personal losses in the last decade and more of life. Even a little or irregular learning would provide some benefits. Inequality is pernicious because it not only reduces benefits from learning at a point in time, but this loss leads to continuous degradation and diminishing returns in the remaining years.

Learning is a mechanism for preventing exclusion and marginalization, both of which have negative outcomes. Exclusion and marginalization have been linked to inequitable social relationships, dependency, decline of wellbeing, diminished participation as a citizen and inability to develop meaningful connections to other generations in society (Silver, 1994). Poorer outcomes of health and quality of life could result in greater use of social programs and larger public expenditures. This heavier use of public services by some has led to the public perception that all people during their entire later years are a burden on other generations.

The United Nations has decried poverty as a violation of human dignity. It lists the negative impacts, which include lack of choices and opportunities, inability to participate effectively in society, personal insecurity, powerlessness and exclusion (United Nations, 1998). As learning poverty has strong interrelationships with many life outcomes, it is associated with multiple deprivations. Social conditions, such as low income, disability and poor living conditions, all exacerbate the lack of access to learning. Learning inequities may concentrate in certain groups or even certain locations. This creates pockets of learning poverty, which results in poor access to information, health care and services, social networks, community participation and cultural life. Concentration of learning poverty among the disadvantaged can start with initial education and continue through life. The social gradient in access to and outcomes of learning launches a vicious circle with a continuing downward spiral in learning. This has long term consequences for health, wellbeing, standard of living and social wellness, all of which are costly for society.

Society gains by lowering learning inequities and nurturing a more informed and knowledgeable population. Losses are high if there is learning deprivation among people in later life. These losses derive from under-developed or unused human capital, lower or poorly informed contributions to society and savings forgone in public costs. Not using human capital reduces economic growth. When everyone contributes at their potential, the long-term value of education and learning continues to pay returns during the years of later life. When the cumulative human capital is not exploited to the fullest for societal benefit, there is an under-developed and unused pool of ability, creating a deficit rather than a 'cognitive surplus' (Halsey, 1961). This lack of efficiency is a major national cost when the unused resource is a large segment of the population. The situation can continue to worsen along with population aging, resulting in perhaps one in five older persons in the population being under-utilized. The costs for subsidizing an unequal society are also an unnecessary expenditure if learning investments can be made instead.

On the other hand, if learning continues through later years, benefits are gained that were not available earlier. As the population in their later years grows, their efforts to supplement the efforts of other generations, fill in gaps and contribute services will provide an additional boost to economic growth. Being healthy in later years will reduce their demands on public and family care. Older citizens will be acknowledged for their value in an age-inclusive society.

5.10 An Inclusive Lifelong Learning System Is a National Investment with High Returns

Learning should be recognized as a lifelong activity. The goals for lifelong learning include the development of diverse skills to develop a sense of mastery and to promote agency, the growth of personal knowledge and aspirations for further learning and the encouragement of curious and critical thinking to push cognition to higher levels. Implementing this requires a lifelong learning system to parallel the trajectory of a learning life course. A lifelong learning system that covers citizens throughout life, including learning options in later life, is a national investment that pays high returns. Providing only recreational learning, which may cater to personal interests and hobbies in later life, means that the later life phase is being undervalued and underserved.

Simple provision of learning options will not by itself result in greater learning during the later years. Success of enabling policies, such as the right to lifelong learning and equal opportunities, depend on individual initiative and responsibility. How well individuals are able to exercise that responsibility for their own benefit depends on their understanding of the value of learning at every year of growth, their learning-to-learn skills and the opportunities to exercise their responsibility. The limiting contextual factors may be strong, so merely removing formal barriers may not change the pattern of learning consumption.

Policies for equality of outcome aim to ensure that people who are disadvantaged can make gains. But equality of opportunities also aims to ensure that everyone has the same opportunities to make those gains. Equality of opportunities has both a de jure and a de facto quality. De jure refers to whether individuals have the same formal options and rights, and de facto refers to the extent to which individuals in reality have them. In other words, the actual options differ across individuals based on context, even if the formal options do not (Sen, 2011). To achieve inclusion in lifelong learning, both the process and the end result are of importance.

Societies will be challenged when adjusting to top-heavy population distributions with a large older segment. The current learning infrastructure cannot be simply extended to include people in their later years. The educational life course must be planned according to the demands of greater longevity. Though aging is a universal phenomenon, human development is very individual. Chronological age does not have universal characteristics nor does it result in equal increments of development. The effects of age are not standardized or consistent during a lifetime or in a given country or context. Although the exact lifetime of individuals cannot be predicted, extending lifelong learning to accommodate prolonged life expectancy requires customization for those in the later stage of life. Achievement depends more on the range of options and personalization of learning than the characteristic of the learner. Training for later life pedagogies based on learning science will be a growing and exciting field because demand from a large share of the population will grow.

5.11 Social Solidarity Includes the Later Years

Understanding the contributing importance of people of different age cohorts and their interrelationships in society builds solidarity across generations. Without such a respectful understanding of the component cohorts, society functions sub-optimally and suffers further fragmentation. It is essential to challenge the outdated narrative describing older persons in the society of the past and to replace it with a realistic but future oriented view. People in their later years can be value-generators for society instead of over-consumers of public services.

How should the citizen spend the extra later years in society? Since people are living longer than ever before, there are no longer models to follow for successful aging. Without a script, life itself becomes the material for creativity in exploring a new vision of productive later life (Fristrup, 2013). Learning is a key component of this biography. Steering life is a way of creating one's own narrative of successful aging. 'Creative aging' (Cohen, 2000) encourages the social construction of contemporary aging by introducing new concepts of successful aging for this generation. The ideal is for society to recognize the value and contribution of the roles people play in their later years, so every generation can envision aging as a constructive part of life.

Creating social norms and symbols related to the aging process and the role and status of people in the later years of life in society is vital. This forms the basis of the social contract. The social contract ensures fairness for all generations and recognizes that each generation will experience the life course in its own time context. The contract influences societal choices involving the value of the later years, especially in raising the potential for a greater longevity dividend.

References

AARP Research. (2021). *2022 tech trends and the 50-plus* (Report). https://www.aarp.org/content/dam/aarp/research/surveys_statistics/technology/2021/2022-technology-trends-older-americans.doi.10.26419-2Fres.00493.001.pdf

Barrett, G. F., & Riddell, W. C. (2019, January). *Ageing and skills: The case of literacy skills* (Discussion paper IZA DP No. 12073). IZA Institute of Labor Economics. https://docs.iza.org/dp12073.pdf

Beckingham, A. C., & Watt, S. (1995). Daring to grow old: Lessons in healthy aging and empowerment. *Educational Gerontology, 21*(5), 479–495. https://www.tandfonline.com/doi/abs/10.1080/0360127950210508

Bjursell, C., Nystedt, P., Björklund, A., & Sternäng, O. (2017). Education level explains participation in work and education later in life. *Educational Gerontology, 43*(10), 511–521. https://doi.org/10.1080/03601277.2017.1357397

Boud, D. (1988). Moving towards autonomy. In D. Boud (Ed.), *Developing student autonomy in learning* (2nd ed., pp. 17–39). Taylor & Francis.

Boud, D., Cohen, R., & Simpson, J. (Eds.). (2001). *Peer learning in higher education: Learning from and with each other*. Routledge.

Brink, S. (2021, September 21). Lifelong learning in later life: Active aging through learning. *EPALE – Electronic Platform for Adult Learning in Europe*. https://epale.ec.europa.eu/en/blog/lifelong-learning-later-life-active-aging-through-learning

Caminotti, E., & Gray, J. (2012). The effectiveness of storytelling on adult learning. *Journal of Workplace Learning, 24*(6), 430–438. https://doi.org/10.1108/13665621211250333

Centre for Educational Research and Innovation. (2007). *Understanding the brain: The birth of a learning science*. OECD Publishing.

Clark, M. C., & Rossiter, M. (2006). "Now the pieces are in place…": Learning through personal storytelling in the adult classroom. *New Horizons in Adult Education & Human Resource Development, 20*(3), 19–33.

Cohen, G. D. (2000). *The creative age: Awakening human potential in the second half of life*. William Morrow.

Cross, K. P. (1981). *Adults as learners: Increasing participation and facilitating learning*. Jossey-Bass.

Davis, H. S. (2013). Discussion as a bridge: Strategies that engage adolescent and adult learning styles in the postsecondary classroom. *Journal of the Scholarship of Teaching and Learning, 13*(1), 68–76. https://scholarworks.iu.edu/journals/index.php/josotl/article/view/2157/3066

de Carteret, P. (2008). Diverse pleasures: Informal learning in community. *Australian Journal of Adult Learning, 48*(3), 502–521. https://ajal.net.au/diverse-pleasures-informal-learning-in-community/

DiSilvestro, F. R. (2013). Continuing higher education and older adults: A growing challenge and golden opportunity. *New Directions for Adult & Continuing Education, 2013*(140), 79–87. https://doi.org/10.1002/ace20076

Findsen, B., & Formosa, M. (2011). *Lifelong learning in later life: A handbook on older adult learning*. Sense Publishers.

Fiocco, A. J., & Yaffe, K. (2010). Defining successful aging: The importance of including cognitive function over time. *Archives of Neurology, 67*(7), 876–880. https://doi.org/10.1001/archneurol.2010.130

Formosa, M. (2002). Critical geragogy: Developing practical possibilities for critical educational gerontology. *Education and Ageing, 17*(1), 73–86. https://www.um.edu.mt/library/oar/handle/123456789/1200

Formosa, M. (2011). Universities of the Third Age: A rationale for transformative education in later life. *Journal of Transformative Education, 8*(3), 197–219. https://doi.org/10.1177/1541344611419857

Fristrup, T. (2013). Craving creativity in later life. In A. Hansen, S. Kling, & J. Šraml González (Eds.), *Creativity, lifelong learning and the ageing population* (Fornvårdaren nr 34) (pp. 56–77). Jamtli Förlag. https://nckultur.org/wp-content/uploads/2013/10/Creativity-lifelong-learning-and-the-ageing-population.pdf

Giddens, A. (1984). *The constitution of society*. University of California Press.

Goddu, K. (2012). Meeting the challenge: Teaching strategies for adult learners. *Kappa Delta Pi Record, 48*(4), 169–173. https://doi.org/10.1080/00228958.2012.734004

Goldberg, E. (2006). *The wisdom paradox: How your mind can grow stronger as your brain grows older*. Avery.

Golding, B., Brown, M., & Foley, A. (2009). Informal learning: A discussion around defining and researching its breadth and importance. *Australian Journal of Adult Learning, 49*(1), 35–56. https://ajal.net.au/informal-learning-a-discussion-around-defining-and-researching-its-breadth-and-importance/

Guinness World Records. (2023, March 5). *Oldest graduate*. https://www.guinnessworldrecords.com/world-records/oldest-graduate

Halsey, A. H. (1961). *Ability and educational opportunity*. OECD Publishing.

Hoffman, P. (2018). An individual differences approach to semantic cognition: Divergent effects of age on representation, retrieval and selection. *Scientific Reports, 8*, Article 8145. https://doi.org/10.1038/s41598-018-26569-0

Illeris, K. (2006). What is special about adult learning? In P. Sutherland & J. Crowther (Eds.), *Lifelong learning: Concepts and contexts* (pp. 15–23). Routledge.

International Labour Organization. (2018). *Global skills trends, training needs and lifelong learning strategies for the future of work. Report prepared by the ILO and OECD for the G20 Employment Working Group.* https://www.ilo.org/wcmsp5/groups/public/%2D%2D-dgreports/%2D%2D-inst/documents/publication/wcms_646038.pdf

Jarvis, P. (2004). *Adult education and lifelong learning: Theory and practice* (3rd ed.). RoutledgeFalmer.

Karge, B. D., Phillips, M. T., Jessee, T., & McCabe, M. (2011). Effective strategies for engaging adult learners. *Journal of College Teaching & Learning, 8*(12), 53–56. https://clutejournals.com/index.php/TLC/article/view/6621/6697

Knowles, M. S. (1975). *Self-directed learning: A guide for learners and teachers*. Association Press.

Knowles, M. S. (1980). *The modern practice of adult education: From pedagogy to andragogy* (Revised and updated). Cambridge Adult Education Co.

Knowles, M. S. and Associates. (1984). *Andragogy in action: Applying modern principles of adult learning*. Jossey-Bass.

Leanos, S., Kürüm, E., Strickland-Hughes, C. M., Ditta, A. S., Nguyen, G., Felix, M., Yum, H., Rebok, G. W., & Wu, R. (2020). The impact of learning multiple real-world skills on cognitive abilities and functional independence in healthy older adults. *The Journals of Gerontology: Series B, 75*(6), 1155–1169. https://doi.org/10.1093/geronb/gbz084

Lindeman, E. C. (1961). *The meaning of adult education*. Harvest House.

Logan, J. R., Ward, R., & Spitze, G. (1992). As old as you feel: Age identity in middle and later life. *Social Forces, 71*(2), 451–467. https://doi.org/10.1093/sf/71.2.451

MacKean, R., & Abbott-Chapman, J. (2011). Leisure activities as a source of informal learning for older people: The role of community-based organisations. *Australian Journal of Adult Learning, 51*(2), 226–247. https://files.eric.ed.gov/fulltext/EJ951995.pdf

Markowsky, G. (2023, January 25). Information theory. In *Encyclopedia Britannica*. https://www.britannica.com/science/information-theory

Martins, R., Simard, F., Provost, J.-S., & Oury, M. (2012). Changes in regional and temporal patterns of activity associated with aging during the performance of a lexical set-shifting task. *Cerebral Cortex, 22*(6), 1395–1406. https://pubmed.ncbi.nlm.nih.gov/21868390/

McNair, S. (2009). *Older people's learning: An action plan*. National Institute of Adult Continuing Education. http://stephenmcnair.uk/wp-content/uploads/2015/07/2009-NIACE-Older-Peoples-Learning-Action-Plan.pdf

McNair, S. (2012). *Older people's learning in 2012: A survey*. National Institute of Adult Continuing Education. https://www.olderpeoplescouncil.org/docs/Older-peoples-learning-in-2012-Summary.pdf

Mezirow, J. (2000). Learning to think like an adult: Core concepts of transformation theory. In J. Mezirow and Associates (Ed.), *Learning as transformation: Critical perspectives on a theory in progress* (pp. 3–33). Jossey-Bass.

Mick, P. T., Hämäläinen, A., Kolisang, L., Pichora-Fuller, M., Phillips, N., Guthrie, D., & Wittich, W. (2021). The prevalence of hearing, vision, and dual sensory loss in older Canadians: An analysis of data from the Canadian Longitudinal Study on Aging. *Canadian Journal on Aging, 40*(1), 1–22. https://psycnet.apa.org/record/2021-19240-001

Milstein, M. (2022). *The age-proof brain: New strategies to improve memory, protect immunity & fight off dementia*. BenBella Books.

OECD. (2002). *Understanding the brain: Towards a new learning science*. https://www.oecd-ilibrary.org/education/understanding-the-brain_9789264174986-en

OECD. (2018). *OECD skills surveys*. https://www.oecd.org/skills/piaac/about/#d.en.481111

Peters, R. (2006). Ageing and the brain. *Postgraduate Medical Journal, 82*(964), 84–88. https://doi.org/10.1136/pgmj.2005.036665

Rathbone, C. H. (1971). *Open education: The informal classroom; a selection of readings that examine the practices and principles of the British infant schools and their American counterparts*. Citation Press.

Rubenson, K. (2011). *Adult learning and education*. Academic.

Rutherford-Hemming, T. (2012). Simulation methodology in nursing education and adult learning theory. *Adult Learning, 23*(3), 129–137. https://journals.sagepub.com/doi/abs/10.1177/1045159512452848

Schaie, K. W. (1984). Midlife influences upon intellectual functioning in old age. *International Journal of Behavioral Development, 7*(4), 463–478. https://doi.org/10.1177/016502548400700405

Schaie, K. W. (1996). *Intellectual development in adulthood: The Seattle Longitudinal Study*. Cambridge University Press.

Schaie, K. W., & Willis, S. L. (2010). The Seattle Longitudinal Study of adult cognitive development. *International Society for the Study of Behavioural Development (ISSBD) Bulletin, 57*(1), 24–29. https://www.ncbi.nlm.nih.gov/pmc/articles/PMC3607395/

Scherling, S. E. (2011). Designing and fostering effective online group projects. *Adult Learning, 22*(2), 13–18. https://doi.org/10.1177/104515951102200202

Schuller, T., & Watson, D. (2009). *Learning through life: Inquiry into the future for lifelong learning* (Summary). National Institute of Adult Continuing Education https://www.cmv-educare.com/wp-content/uploads/2015/12/schuller.pdf

Sen, A. (2011). *The idea of justice*. Belknap Press.

Shih, M. J., Pittinsky, T. L., & Ho, G. C. (2012). Stereotype boost: Positive outcomes from the activation of positive stereotypes. In M. Inzlicht & T. Schmader (Eds.), *Stereotype threat: Theory, process, and application* (pp. 141–143). Oxford University Press.

Silver, H. (1994). Social exclusion and social solidarity: Three paradigms. *International Labour Review, 133*(5–6), 531–578. https://www.academia.edu/16848270/Social_Exclusion_and_Social_Solidarity_Three_Paradigms

Smith, L. B., & Thelen, E. (1994). *A dynamic systems approach to the development of cognition and action*. MIT Press.

Statistics Canada. (2021, June 22). Canadian Internet Use Survey, 2020. *The Daily*. https://www150.statcan.gc.ca/n1/en/daily-quotidien/210622/dq210622b-eng.pdf?st=TF0MQPPd

Statistics Canada. (2022). *Census family status and household living arrangements, household type of person, age group and gender: Canada, provinces and territories, census metropolitan areas and census agglomerations* (Table 98-10-0134-01). https://doi.org/10.25318/9810013401-eng

Stats NZ. (2020, October 8). *Cruise ship traveller and expenditure statistics: Year ended June, 2020*. https://www.stats.govt.nz/information-releases/cruise-ship-traveller-and-expenditure-statistics-year-ended-june-2020/

Steele, C. M., & Aronson, J. (1995). Stereotype threat and the intellectual test performance of African Americans. *Journal of Personality and Social Psychology, 69*(5), 797–811. https://doi.org/10.1037/0022-3514.69.5.797

Taylor, E. W. (1998). *The theory and practice of transformative learning: A critical review* (Information series no. 374). ERIC Clearing House on Adult, Career, and Vocational Education. https://files.eric.ed.gov/fulltext/ED423422.pdf

Tight, M. (2003). *Key concepts in adult education and training*. Routledge.

Tough, A. (1971). *The adult's learning projects: A fresh approach to theory and practice in adult learning*. Ontario Institute for Studies in Education.

UNESCO. (n.d.). *TVETipedia glossary*. International Centre for Technical and Vocational Education and Training. https://unevoc.unesco.org/home/TVETipedia+Glossary

United Nations. (1998, May 20). *Statement of commitment for action to eradicate poverty adopted by Administrative Committee on Coordination* (Press release ECOSOC/5759). Economic and Social Council. https://press.un.org/en/1998/19980520.eco5759.html

Ventura-Merkel, C., & Lidoff, L. (1983). *Community planning for intergenerational programming* (Program innovation in aging) (Vol. VIII). National Council on Aging.

Weinstein, C. E., Jung, J., & Acee, T. W. (2010). Learning strategies. In P. Peterson, E. Baker, & B. McGaw (Eds.), *International encyclopedia of education* (3rd ed., pp. 323–329). https://doi.org/10.1016/B978-0-08-044894-7.00497-8

Wenger, E., McDermott, R., & Snyder, W. M. (2002). *Cultivating communities of practice: A guide to managing knowledge*. Harvard Business School Press.

Whitbourne, S. K., & Montepare, J. M. (2017). What's holding us back? Ageism in higher education. In T. D. Nelson (Ed.), *Ageism: Stereotyping and prejudice against older persons* (2nd ed., pp. 263–290). MIT Press. https://doi.org/10.7551/mitpress/10679.003.0015

World Health Organization. (2020, October 26). *Healthy ageing and functional ability*. Questions and answers. https://www.who.int/news-room/questions-and-answers/item/healthy-ageing-and-functional-ability

Chapter 6
Understanding the Longevity Dividend

The living generations of today are experiencing a society unlike any before where there are more older people than children and youth. The size of the older cohorts will grow larger than they have before because of growing life expectancy. Longevity is a reality, and both individuals and societies have to be ready for the demand for longer purposeful lives for citizens and for continuing wellbeing and prosperity in mature societies.

6.1 Longevity Impacts Population Structure

The population age distribution patterns of a country at a particular time can be described by population pyramids, which portray the number or percentages of men and women of younger age cohorts at the bottom and of older cohorts in the population at the top. In this century many countries are undergoing a change in population structure. Greater longevity is changing the shape of the population pyramid, with each shape marking the stage attained in the population aging process.

6.1.1 Expansive Stage

Countries with a high birthrate and a short life expectancy have large cohorts of children and small cohorts of older people. This results in the classic pyramid shaped population distribution seen in Fig. 6.1, called the expansive stage (Saroha, 2018). In most countries this population distribution was generally prevalent when the education systems for children were designed. Economic growth was likely to be low, as the adult workforce was small compared to the number of children.

S. Brink, *The Longevity Dividend*, International Perspectives on Aging 39,
https://doi.org/10.1007/978-3-031-35335-2_6

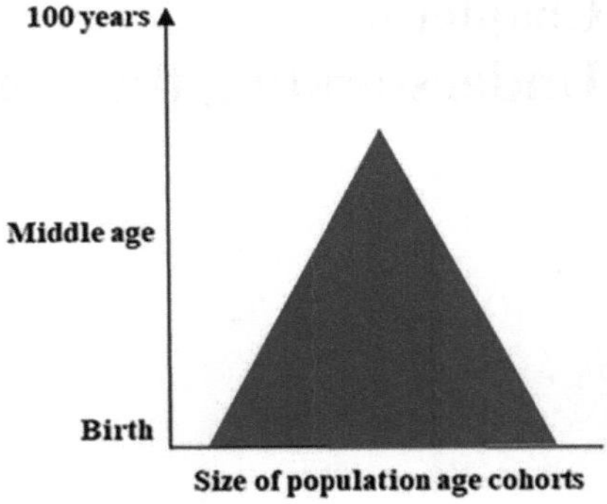

Fig. 6.1 Population pyramid in the expansive stage with many children and few older people

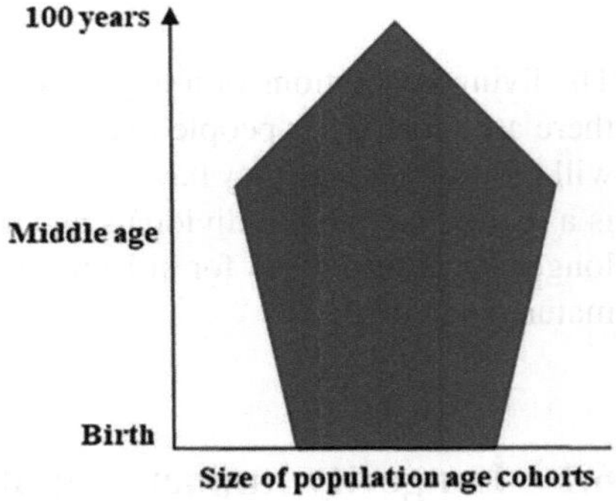

Fig. 6.2 Population pyramid with a working age bulge and a low birth rate

6.1.2 Working Age Bulge

If populations have had high birthrates a few decades prior, and those children have now reached prime working age, there is likely to be a working age bulge. This bulge is often accompanied by a lower birthrate, resulting in a population pyramid that is wider in the middle, where the large middle-aged cohorts are located and narrower at the bottom due to fewer children (Saroha, 2018). Economies tend to grow faster because of the larger contributions by the working age population in the labour market. More people may be able to afford higher education (Fig. 6.2).

6.1.3 Population Aging

When the population has high life expectancy along with a low birthrate, the population pyramid is top heavy with large older cohorts. There are small cohorts of centenarians at the very top and a small base of child cohorts. The pyramid can assume a jar shape as in Fig. 6.3 (Saroha, 2018). The imbalance is usually measured by the dependency ratio, or the total number of the population too young or too old

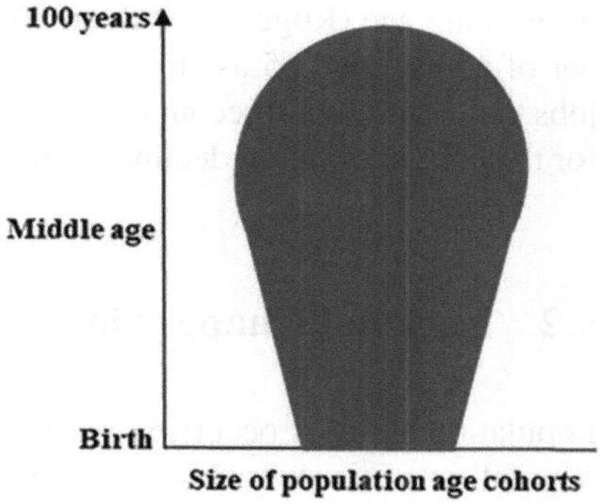

Fig. 6.3 Population pyramid with large old cohorts and small cohorts of working age and children

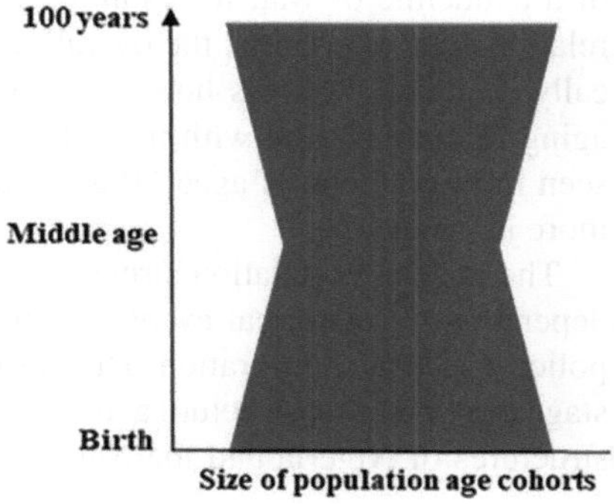

Fig. 6.4 Population pyramid with cohorts of older people and children larger than working age cohorts

to work, divided by the number of the population 15–65 years (people of working age). A high dependency ratio indicates a high burden of support on workers in the labour force for dependents, seen in purely labour market terms. Economic growth and incomes may be higher, but the public discourse has focused on higher public costs for health care, income security and social services for the older cohorts. These concerns generate interest in stimulating a higher birthrate with generous support to families with children and other child-friendly policies as well as incentives to encourage people to work longer.

6.1.4 Shrinking Workforce Compared to Young and Old Cohorts

Continued increases in life expectancy results in larger cohorts of older people and stable birthrates of children compared to cohorts of working age. This can generate the hourglass shaped population pyramid in Fig. 6.4 (Saroha, 2018). For example, over the decade 2010–2020, the growth of the non-working age population of children 0–14 and people 65 and older in the United States outpaced the growth of those of working age (Rogers & Wilder, 2020). By 2020, there was about the same number of adults aged 65 as children under 18 years. Longer working careers in good jobs can contribute to economic growth and a high rate of savings. The total costs for the care of children declines, but they receive good quality education.

6.2 National Changes in Population Structure

Population aging is occurring worldwide, but national experience with changes in population structure varies. The population structure of a given country has its own growth pattern, varying with its history and the timing of particular issues (impact of a pandemic or war, for example). Though these national events affect the size relationships of cohorts, the overall direction of change is rarely changed dramatically. Figure 6.5 shows how the population structure of Finland was affected by aging in combination with its history of events. The effect of population aging is seen in larger cohorts aged 90 and over and in the population structure becoming more jar shaped.

The shift in population structure occurs at different rates and at different times depending on historical events, birth rate, growth in average life expectancy and policies such as immigration. This results in large variation among countries in their stage of population structure at a particular time. Figure 6.6 contrasts the population structures of Nigeria and the Netherlands in 2019. Nigeria's large population was

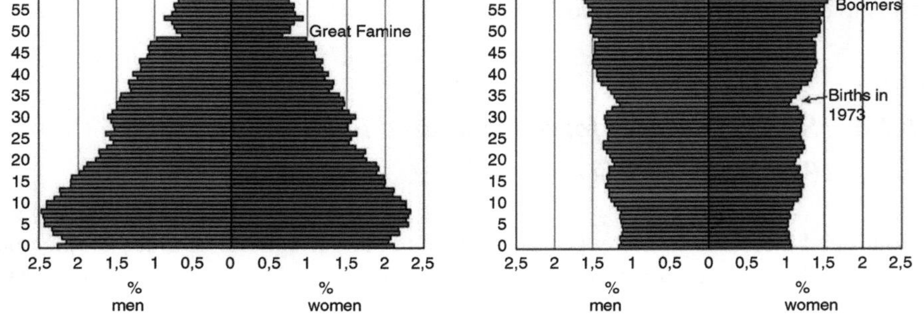

Fig. 6.5 Population pyramids of Finland in 1917 and 2006. (Reproduced from Population development in independent Finland – greying Baby Boomers by Statistics Finland (2007, Fig. 1). CC BY Attribution 4 International)

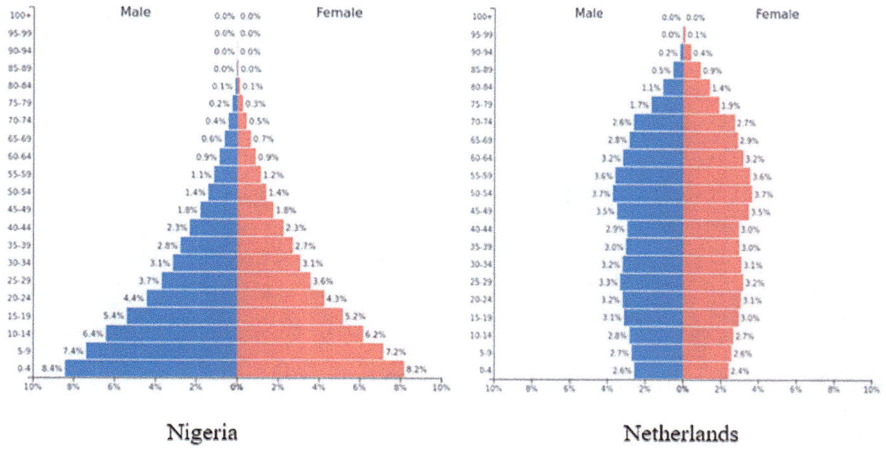

Fig. 6.6 Population pyramids of Nigeria and the Netherlands, 2019. Selected at PopulationPyramid.net (2023). (CC BY 3.0 IGO)

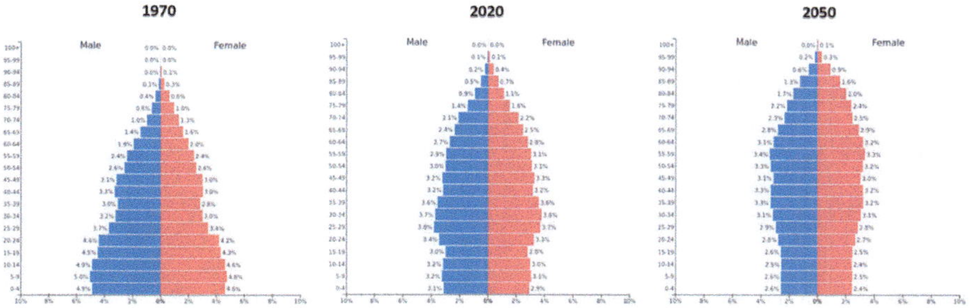

Fig. 6.7 Population pyramids of Australia, 1970, 2020, 2050. Selected at PopulationPyramid.net (2023). (CC BY 3.0 IGO)

still in the expansive stage with its population structure in the pyramid shape. The population structure of the Netherlands displayed the effect of population aging having occurred over some time. The rate of change in structure has consequences for a country's time available to plan for population aging.

The timing of the transition of population structure over time depends on the country. There is no set time progression. However, statistical projection of specific population distributions can indicate when a country should act to take advantage of the opportunities linked to population aging. Figures 6.7, 6.8 and 6.9 show selected examples of countries with different population growth patterns over time.

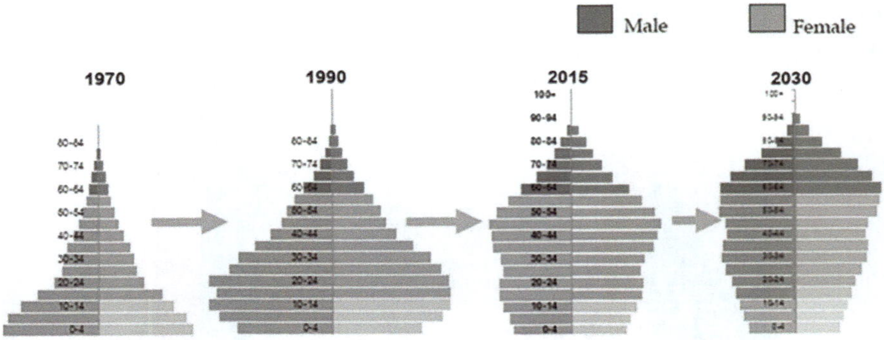

Fig. 6.8 Population pyramids of Thailand, 1970, 1990, 2015, 2030. (Reproduced from Prospects and contexts of demographic transitions in Thailand by Prasartkul et al. (2019, p. 16) with permission from Journal of Population and Social Studies)

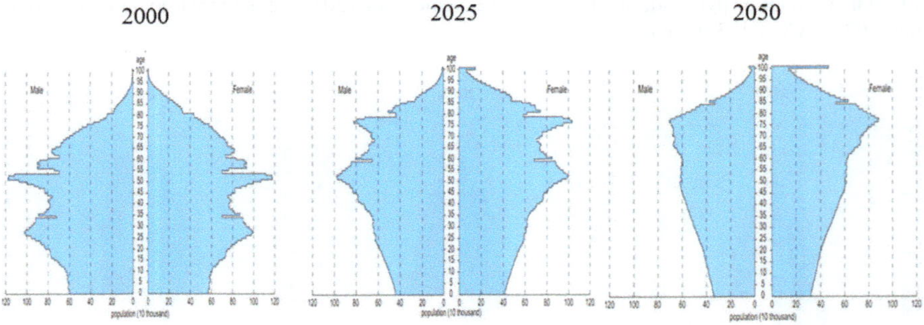

Fig. 6.9 Population pyramids of Japan, 2000, 2025, 2050. (Reproduced from Population projections for Japan: 2001–2050 by National Institute of Population and Social Security Research, 2002)

6.3 Demographic Transitions

The population pyramids shown indicate that population shifts can be considerable. As a society prepares for the period after the start of the transition, there is time for individual and collective transformation. A demographic dividend is the potential economic growth, over and above related costs, that can occur only during such shifts in the population's age structure. The gains from a population transition depends on how a society manages the opportunities and costs related to the changes in age structure (United Nations Population Fund, 2016). The two demographic transitions thus far – one related to lower fertility rates and one to greater life expectancy – can be accompanied by strategic societal action to realize the potential of the growing population segment and to invest in it to realize a sizeable societal gain. While the demographic transitions can be predicted in advance, the potential individual and collective benefits that can be realized depend on the accompanying societal changes and are not easily predicted.

The populations of developed countries appear to have gone through a first demographic transition from a combination of high fertility and high mortality to low fertility and low mortality. The first indication of the high fertility was when most newborns survived. Countries that benefited from this bonanza were able to provide these children with good health and education. This societal investment resulted in a large, well-educated young labour force as they matured into adulthood. Generally, this generation grew up in relatively peaceful and prosperous times. The larger adult cohort contributed to their own economic wellbeing, the advancement of the standard of living and the development of their countries. They were able to pay back to society throughout their lives through labour force participation, good health and savings. They nurtured and educated their children, further contributing to society's development and progress. Although a once-only opportunity, of a short-term and transitory nature (a few decades), the transition provided a temporary bonus, sometimes called the youth dividend (Lee & Mason, 2006). However, the benefit is not automatic – it depends on the policies chosen and their effectiveness.

The second demographic transition is the shift from a population with a high proportion of children to one with a high proportion of older people as life expectancy increases. The population becomes top heavy with large cohorts of well-educated adults of working and older ages. As workers with high skills and long experience work longer, the productivity of the work force rises. While the growth of the working population slows, older cohorts accumulate wealth, grow their investments and save for their future retirement. Although aged cohorts are no longer in the workforce, they continue to generate consumer demand and make valuable contributions to society. These cumulative contributions can push the national trajectory of growth and progress upwards during the population transition. The value of this dividend is determined by the public and private choices made in order to benefit from the increase in longevity. It is thus described as the longevity dividend.

6.4 Are the Demographic Dividends Worth the Effort?

Countries are at different points in the growth and age distribution of their populations. Because the demographic shift can be predicted in advance, making too late an effort to benefit from it has been described as kicking an already open door. Each country has its own population growth pattern and has to find a working strategy of its own to gain from the demographic dividends. For instance, countries that grew richer before they grew older could design policies to amplify the benefits. Those that had strong economic growth during the years of the working age bulge could benefit from having an older population with savings for spending in their later years. The value of the demographic dividend depends on the context, the predominant cohorts, the balance between the costs and benefits to society and the length of time over which contributions to society are made. Typically, the gains from the

Table 6.1 Demographic dividends: Contribution to growth in GDP per effective consumer

	Contribution to growth in GDP per effective consumer			
Regions	First dividend	Second dividend	Total	Actual growth in GDP per effective consumer
Industrial economies	0.34	0.69	1.03	2.25
East and Southeast Asia	0.59	1.31	1.90	4.32
South Asia	0.10	0.69	0.79	1.88
Latin America	0.62	1.08	1.70	0.94
Sub-Saharan Africa	−0.09	0.17	0.08	0.06
Middle East and North Africa	0.51	0.70	1.21	1.10

Note: Actual growth in GDP per effective consumer, 1970–2000, in percent per year. Number of effective consumers is the number of consumers weighted for age variation in consumption needs Reproduced from Demographic transition and demographic dividends in developed and developing countries by Mason (2007, Table 3) with permission from A. Mason

second longevity dividend are greater than the first youth dividend. The longevity dividend is also likely to be longer lasting, since life expectancy is still growing and larger proportions of the older cohorts are living longer.

The size of effect of the demographic dividend on a society's economic growth can vary. Some countries have been more successful than others in achieving economic gains from the demographic dividends. Table 6.1 illustrates the effects measured over a 30-year period.

Between 1970 and 2000, both the first and second dividends had mainly positive effects. The economic contribution of the second dividend, through increased capital accumulation, was larger than that of the first dividend, and the calculated combined effect of both dividends was as high as 1.9% a year in East and Southeast Asia. In that region, the demographic dividends contributed 44% of the actual growth per economic consumer. Latin America was less successful in exploiting the opportunity presented by demographic dividends. In Latin America, the dividends could have contributed economic growth of 1.7% per year, but actual growth was only 0.9% (Lee & Mason, 2006, 2010).

6.5 Understanding the Potential of the Longevity Dividend

The second demographic dividend was first named the 'longevity dividend' in 2006 by Olshansky and colleagues, noting the economic savings that resulted from healthy aging during longer lives (Olshansky, 2013; Olshansky et al., 2016). The longevity dividend is the economic growth and social progress, over and above related costs, generated by longer and growing life expectancy. It occurs only once because the increasing life expectancy shifts the population composition from one containing a large proportion of children to a large proportion of older people, and it is unlikely to revert. In this altered population structure, large numbers of adults with knowledge and skills can collectively contribute more to society than before. (Chapter 3 above describes the productive contributions of people in the later years of life). Their contributions can be considered productive as they increase growth, reduce costs or foster social progress.

The contributions can be maximized by societal choices that include older people in the knowledge pool and increase human capital through lifelong learning. As a larger proportion of citizens live longer than before, their total contributions of societal value rise over their lifetime, compared to expected contributions based on smaller numbers of citizens with shorter life expectancy. This once-only transition in population structure, driven by longer lives, raises the national trajectory of economic growth and social progress. Once the population distribution is stabilized, the rate of growth slows but retains the benefit of this potentially large one-time increase (Government of Singapore, 2023). Figure 6.10 illustrates the once-only nature of the longevity dividend. While the societal benefit has traditionally been measured in economic terms by increases in the Gross Domestic Product, the gains are potentially broader.

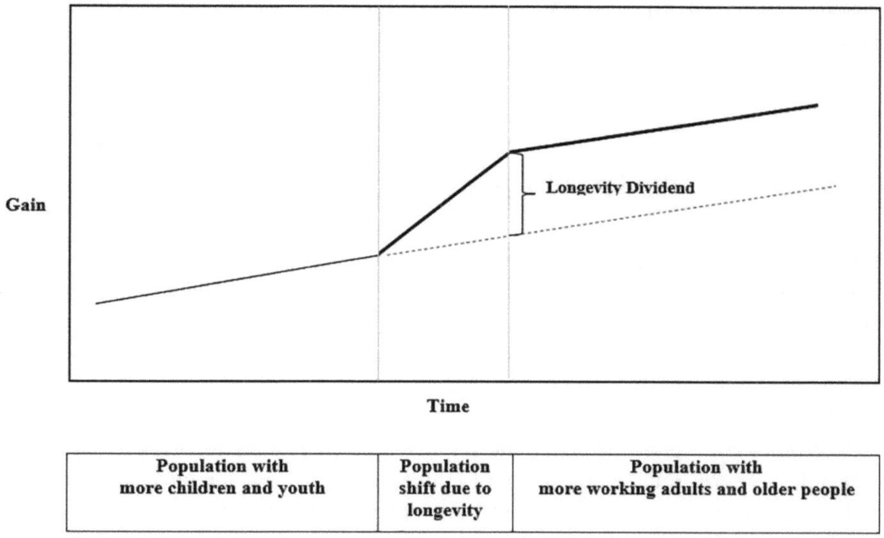

Fig. 6.10 The longevity dividend is a one-time gain, which can be increased by choices made during the population transition. (Author's elaboration, 2023)

6.6 Recognizing the Progress of the Population Transition and Its Potential

There are more people aged 65 and over alive today than ever before. Older persons constitute a large proportion of the population globally. This aging phenomenon of the population was unimaginable before – a significant social transformation of the twenty-first century (Department of Economic and Social Affairs, 2015). Despite projections of change, societies are slow to prepare for the consequences even as life expectancies continue to increase rapidly in many countries. In 1980, Sweden had the largest percentage (16%) of people 65 years and over. Japan led with 30% of people aged 65 and over in 2021 but in 2050, China and Hong Kong are projected to have over 40% (Department of Economic and Social Affairs, 2023). By 2050 one in six people in the world will be over 65 years, an increase from one in ten in 2022. Since 1840, life expectancy at birth has risen about 3 months with each passing year (Easterbrook, 2014). Life expectancy at birth in Sweden in 1840 was 45 years for women; currently it is 83 years. If about 3 months continue to be added with each passing year, American life expectancy at birth will be 88 years by the middle of this century. By the end of the century, it will be 100 years.

Longevity is no longer the exception but a normal feature of life. Those aged over 65 can form a quarter of the population in several countries. For instance, by 2030 older persons are expected to form more than 25% of the populations of Europe and North America (Department of Economic and Social Affairs, 2015). This population segment can have both economic clout and powerful policy influence.

6.7 A Finite Window of Opportunity That Occurs Just Once

The multiple characteristics of this population transition makes it a one-time opportunity. Why? It is unlikely that populations in countries will repeat the birthrate and mortality conditions of either the first or second transitions in the foreseeable future. The numerous and simultaneous policy changes and investments have to be made before the finite window gradually closes as the transition ends and conditions stabilize.

The older cohorts of the next generation share some characteristics with the current older cohorts, such as the level of education. However, the current generation had some advantages, compared to the next generation. They started working earlier and were able to build their net worth through longer and careful saving and investments in homes, facilitated by living in peaceful and prosperous times.

The choices societies make related to the increase in older citizens in their population affect the gains from the longevity dividend. As shown in Table 6.1, there can be considerable variation in the gains among regions in the world. Societies that intentionally choose to take advantage of the transition by making strategic choices can enhance the longevity dividend more than societies that do not.

Once a reformed suite of policies is cemented during the transition, they can ensure the flow of benefits to form the longevity dividend. They will also ensure that development and progress after the transition will continue from the culmination of the gains from the longevity dividend rather than starting from a lower point (Fig. 6.10). Though the rate of increase in subsequent gains may not be as high as during the transition, the investments made to accommodate population aging can allow progress to continue at rates that would not have been achieved otherwise.

6.8 Strategic Choices Enhance the Longevity Dividend

Given the factors that affect the longevity dividend, there are two key ways to increase the gains. First, societies can take strategic action to increase the total productive contributions that benefit society. Steps can be taken to improve healthy aging by encouraging positive health practices, ensuring self-care through life, providing lifelong accessible health care and mitigating illnesses or disability. This can increase the number of active years in a lifetime during which such productive contributions can be made. If the time given to total productive contributions can be increased during each individual's lifetime, the cumulative national total can be increased.

Second, investing in a lifelong learning system improves not only the life outcomes and quality of life of individuals, but it also enables them to improve the quantity and quality of their contributions in terms of timeliness, appropriateness and added value. They are aging in a world that is transforming in multiple ways during their lifetime. Lifelong learning enables them to understand the context, appraise needs, and choose the best options. They will know how to apply the appropriate knowledge and skills for decisions and actions taken for personal or societal benefit. Thus, lifelong learning increases the quantity and quality of their contributions of value to society. It could be more strategic for policy planners and decision makers to look not only at the age dependency ratio (the sum of the population under 15 years and the population 65 and over relative to the working age population 15–64 years) but to consider the combined adult population (16–100 years) and their potential human capital and societal contributions.

6.9 The Foundations for Lifelong Learning Have Been Laid

Education, training and learning have become necessities in modern life. The proportion of the world population without any education will decline drastically. For instance, the global illiteracy rate fell from 44% in 1950 to 14% in 2016 (Roser & Ortiz-Ospina, 2016). Global action to provide schooling to all children has resulted in higher literacy and education attainment in the population of most countries. There will be differences in the education levels among citizens of a country, but so long as the goal of making education universal and ensuring that public expenditures are adequate, the average education attainment level of every country is likely to grow.

The investments in education result in a better educated populace. The mean years of schooling globally is projected to increase steadily from 8.6 years in 2010 to 12.1 years in 2050 and further to 14.1 years in 2100 (Samir & Lutz, 2017). High school graduation rates are high in developed countries with universal public education. For example, in 2017 high school graduates composed 99% of the population in Finland, 98% in Japan, 97% in New Zealand, and 93% in Korea (OECD, 2017).

A generational change can be expected in the human capital gains in society through education for a greater number of people. Post-secondary education used to be available to a minority of the population. In the 1970s, globally there were only about 700 million people with secondary or post-secondary education, but this figure is predicted to increase tenfold by 2100 (Roser & Ortiz-Ospina, 2016). On average about 40% of workers aged 25–64 in OECD countries had tertiary education in 2021 (OECD, 2021). Most countries will in the years to come show a noticeable increase in the population with higher education and a decrease in those with only basic education (Table 6.2).

The impacts of rising education levels are immense. Schooling provides a foundation of knowledge and literacy skills, which increases the capacity to learn, consume, evaluate and apply information after graduation. People with more education tend to seek further education more than those with less. Education opens opportunities for employment, income security and better standards of living throughout life. Societies with educated residents can anticipate higher expectations and participation by an involved and active citizenry.

Table 6.2 Populations aged 15 years and over with tertiary education shows major increases, selected countries, 1970 and 2050

	Adult population with tertiary education	
Country	1970 (%)	2050 (%)
Canada	10.9	46.1
Colombia	2.1	30.3
Japan	8.5	55.8
South Korea	3.2	51.7
Thailand	1.4	31.8
United Kingdom	8.5	38.8

Source: Roser and Ortiz-Ospina (2013). Creative commons CC BY

6.10 The Combined Effect of Rising Education and Longevity

Just decades ago, children aspired to have more education than their parents. Ambitious parents went into debt to send their children to good universities at home or abroad. There have always been intra-cohort and inter-cohort differences in educational attainment, but they are likely weakening as education becomes more accessible and less related to age or generation. Data from the European Union shows how the older population not only grows in size over time but is also more educated (Fig. 6.11).

Today's large population of older cohorts in many countries has a good education and have had valuable careers, contributing to their own progress, their profession, their employers and the country. As these educated cohorts approach age 65 they are more willing to work longer or to start a second career. For example, in the United States, 31% of people who were still in the labour force past age 65 had earned a master's degree or higher, while just 15% and 25% were, respectively, those with only a high-school diploma or a bachelor's degree (Schramm, 2018). Growth in educational attainment starts a virtuous spiral towards larger numbers with more education among the older cohorts. Those with better education tend to enjoy better health and live longer. They are better able to age successfully, contribute to society and be part of a national cognitive reserve.

6.11 Successful Population Aging Requires Culture Change

Today's understanding of the effects of population aging cannot be based on the past. Still, the aging of populations is often dreaded because existing culture continues to see a high birth rate and a large labour force as fundamental. The impact of baby boomer generations attaining old age, with a relatively large number of older people dependent on a smaller generation of workers aged 15–64 years, was thought to be dramatic and catastrophic. Population aging and longevity were considered negative phenomena. Doomsday predictions and gloomy prognostications with such terms as the 'silver tsunami' (Maples, 2007) dominated the public discourse.

To live and prosper in a society where more people are old is different from past human history, where most people were young and more educated than the old in society. The youth culture is now less valid. Aging has to be re-defined as a social construct, and the role of older people in society has to be rethought at the same time as the population transition proceeds. The concept of aging should perhaps apply to the life course, or the journey through the life span may need a different vocabulary that transcends aging.

Culture has to accommodate new ways of thinking about the large older segment of the population. Not only are people living longer but they are healthier and more

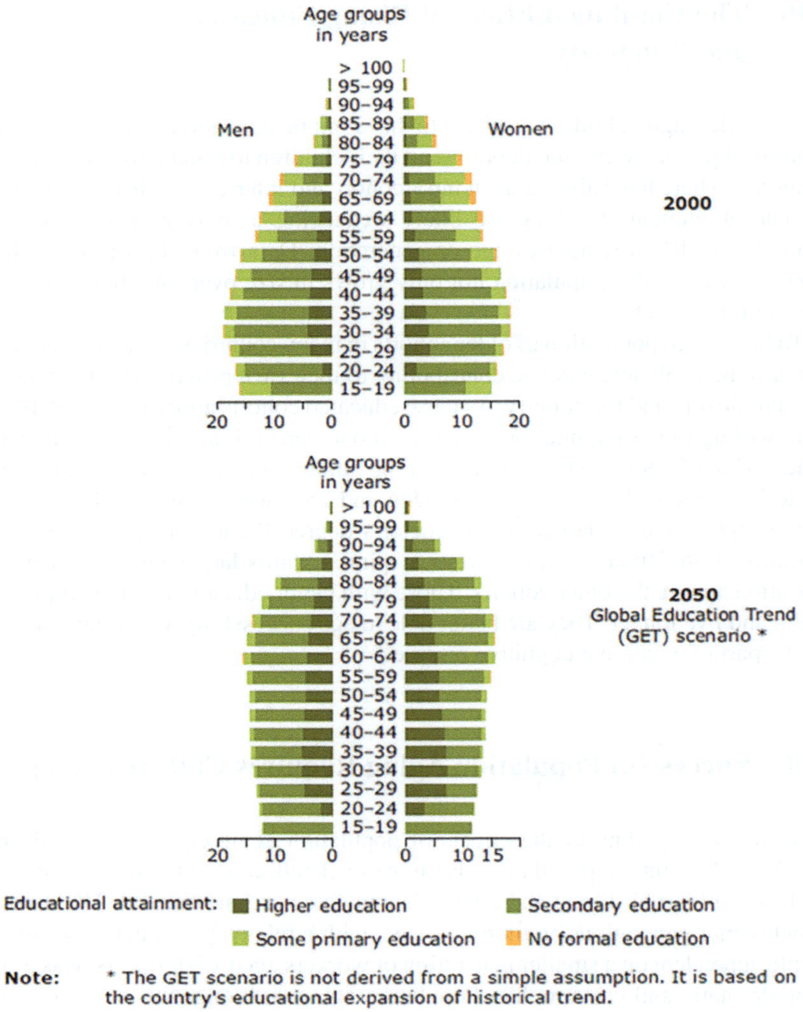

Fig. 6.11 The older population will be more educated with time. Population by age, sex and educational attainment, European Union, 2000 and 2050. (Reproduced from European Environment Agency, 2011, Fig. 1.4a. CC BY 2.5 DK)

actively engaged for longer parts of their lives. It makes no sense to misrepresent a quarter of the population that although old is generally active and healthy. Many age-related conditions that once impeded active living are now avoided, delayed or diminished by treatment or supporting devices. When integrated well into society, this large population segment can be a positive force with their accumulated knowledge and life experience.

The relationship of people in later life with younger generations has to be reformulated. Rather than considering the older generation as dependent on people of working age, the mutual exchanges of benefits must be recognized. Contributions and intergenerational transfers involve almost everything, such as genes, governance, justice, infrastructure, wealth and culture, to name a few. Such contributions minimize decline during transitions and ensure progress through intergenerationally shared benefits.

Culture is a way of life which can build solidarity to work together towards a shared destiny. A society where the population mix is changing can modify its policies but a change in culture is required for policy acceptance. It can be difficult to change an ingrained narrative that a large older population is a burden. Society must nonetheless reorganize its functioning to equip all its members for more years of active living. Social reconstruction of the concept of aging is slow and new social construction is even slower. An alternative perspective frames a long-lived older population as an opportunity for progress by creating value from the population shift (Jarvis, 2008). A society that is no longer characterized by an age-segmented culture will make strategic choices based on a life span that can generate long term benefits arising from the longevity dividend.

6.12 The Sparks That Ignite Culture Change

The responsibility for generating culture change as longevity increases is shared between a country as a polity and its individual citizens. Social choices are reflected by key democratic decisions to pursue a package of signaling policies. Signaling policies convey information on changes in shared beliefs and validate changes in accepted norms. In the package of signaling policies are those that address lifelong phenomena, including the later life component of a longer lifetime and equitable health care that meets the specific needs of particular age groups from birth to death. The signaling policies are also those that highlight public investments specifically for the wellbeing of citizens during the years of later life, such as support for lifelong learning also in the later years. The total package thus signals the interdependence of all ages and the perceived status of later life in societal culture.

The responsibility of citizens is to respond to the signals as individuals and as society. Signals help individuals to construct their identity in a desirable society where everyone can age well throughout life. The signals reinforce in a concrete and visible way, for citizens individually and collectively, the value of people during the entire life course.

These actions will lead to a culture for a mature society.

References

Department of Economic and Social Affairs. (2015). *World population ageing 2015 – Highlights* (ST/ESA/SER.A/368). United Nations. https://www.un.org/en/development/desa/population/publications/pdf/ageing/WPA2015_Highlights.pdf

Department of Economic and Social Affairs. (2023). *World Social Report 2023: Leaving no one behind in an ageing world.* United Nations. https://www.un.org/development/desa/dspd/wp-content/uploads/sites/22/2023/01/2023wsr-fullreport.pdf

Easterbrook, G. (2014, October). What happens when we all live to 100? *The Atlantic*. https://www.theatlantic.com/magazine/archive/2014/10/what-happens-when-we-all-live-to-100/379338/

European Environment Agency. (2011). *The European environment – State and outlook 2010: Assessment of global megatrends.* https://www.eea.europa.eu/soer/2010/europe-and-the-world/megatrends

Government of Singapore. (2023, February 15). *SkillsFuture*. https://www.skillsfuture.gov.sg/

Jarvis, P. (2008). *Democracy, lifelong learning and the learning society: Active citizenship in a late modern age*. Routledge.

Lee, R., & Mason, A. (2006). What is the demographic dividend? *Finance and Development, 43*(3). International Monetary Fund. https://www.imf.org/external/pubs/ft/fandd/2006/09/index.htm

Lee, R., & Mason, A. (2010). Fertility, human capital, and economic growth over the demographic transition. *European Journal of Population, 26*, 159–182. https://doi.org/10.1007/s10680-009-9186-x

Maples, M. F. (2007). *Spirituality, wellness and the "Silver Tsunami": Implications for counseling*. https://www.counseling.org/resources/library/vistas/2007-V-online-MSWord-files/Maples.pdf

Mason, A. (2007). Demographic transition and demographic dividends in developed and developing countries. In *Department of Economic and Social Affairs, United Nations Expert Group Meeting on Social and Economic Implications of Changing Population Age Structures* (ESA/P/WP.201, pp. 81–101). https://www.un.org/en/development/desa/population/events/pdf/expert/9/full_report.pdf

National Institute of Population and Social Security Research. (2002). *Population projections for Japan: 2001–2050*. https://www.ipss.go.jp/pp-newest/e/ppfj02/ppfj02.pdf

OECD. (2017). *Education at a glance 2017: OECD indicators*. OECD Publishing. https://doi.org/10.1787/eag-2017-en

OECD. (2021). *Population with tertiary education* (Indicator) [Data set]. https://doi.org/10.1787/0b8f90e9-en

Olshansky, S. J. (2013). Articulating the case for the longevity dividend. *Public Policy & Aging Report, 23*(4), 3–6. https://www.afar.org/images/uploads/general/Olshansky_LongevityDividend.pdf

Olshansky, S. J., Martin, G. M., & Kirkland, J. L. (2016). *Aging: The longevity dividend.* Cold Spring Harbor Laboratory Press.

PopulationPyramid.net. (2023). *Population pyramids of the world from 1950 to 2100* [Data portal]. https://www.populationpyramid.net/

Prasartkul, P., Thaweesit, S., & Chuanwan, S. (2019). Prospects and contexts of demographic transitions in Thailand. *Journal of Population and Social Studies, 27*(1), 1–22. https://so03.tci-thaijo.org/index.php/jpss/article/view/119341/113993

Rogers, L., & Wilder, K. (2020, June 25). *Shift in working-age population relative to older and younger Americans*. United States Census Bureau. https://www.census.gov/library/stories/2020/06/working-age-population-not-keeping-pace-with-growth-in-older-americans.html

Roser, M., & Ortiz-Ospina, E. (2013). *Tertiary education*. OurWorldInData.org [Based on data from International Institute for Applied Systems Analysis]. https://ourworldindata.org/tertiary-education

Roser, M., & Ortiz-Ospina, E. (2016). *Global education*. OurWorldInData.org [Based on OECD and UNESCO data]. https://ourworldindata.org/global-education

Samir, K. C., & Lutz, W. (2017). The human core of the shared socioeconomic pathways: Population scenarios by age, sex and level of education for all countries to 2100. *Global Environmental Change, 42*(January), 181–192. https://doi.org/10.1016/j.gloenvcha.2014.06.004

Saroha, J. (2018). Types and significance of population pyramids. *World Wide Journal of Multidisciplinary Research and Development, 4*(4), 59–69. http://wwjmrd.com/upload/types-and-significance-of-population-pyramids_1523552342.pdf

Schramm, J. (2018, September). *An aging labor force and the challenges of 65+ jobseekers.* AARP Public Policy Institute. https://www.aarp.org/content/dam/aarp/ppi/2018/09/an-aging-labor-force-and-the-challenges-of-sixty-five-plus-jobseekers.pdf

Statistics Finland. (2007). *Population development in independent Finland – Greying Baby Boomers*. Finland 1917–2007. https://www.stat.fi/tup/suomi90/joulukuu_en.html

United Nations Population Fund. (2016). *Demographic dividend.* https://www.unfpa.org/demographic-dividend#NaN

Chapter 7
Societal Choices Enhance the Longevity Dividend

The magnitude of the longevity dividend depends on the strategic choices societies make when experiencing population aging. The strategy involves systemic thinking to generate inter-related policies. Choices that transform society are easier to implement if cultural change creates an encouraging policy environment and increases popular support. Countries that developed into advanced economies had a smoother path to embracing population aging because most aging citizens were relatively economically comfortable. People in such societies adapted to longer lives because their education and work lives prepared them for active aging with a longer health span and they chose to use their knowledge and skills to be active participants in society.

A primary strategy to enlarge the longevity dividend is to increase the total contributions made by individuals that benefit society. Productive contributions can add to economic growth, decrease waste and reduce costs and encourage social development. People can start contributing to society as early as their teenage years and continue to the end of life. Because of increased longevity, the productive years during which such contributions can be made are more numerous. The number of hours of contribution in each year can vary during the life course, but the number of hours per year may be higher in later life, because older people have both time and the applicable knowledge and skills. Their efforts increase the total annual number of hours of productive contributions to society. For instance, older people could live active lives and volunteer more hours.

The second strategy is to increase the quality of the contribution, thus increasing their value to society. The greater diversity of ways in which older persons can simultaneously make multiple contributions and their greater effectiveness enhance quality. Lifelong learning can increase both the quantity and quality of the lifetime contributions of citizens to society. Depending on the prevailing culture, countries may choose policies to adapt to greater longevity and invest early in order to augment the longevity dividend.

S. Brink, *The Longevity Dividend*, International Perspectives on Aging 39,
https://doi.org/10.1007/978-3-031-35335-2_7

7.1 Societies Can Benefit from the Experience of Countries that Aged Faster or Earlier

The initial national policy responses to population aging were defensive, focused on reducing the public expenditure on health and pensions by lowering public health allocations and reducing economic assistance and services to older people. As societies began to adapt, the societal changes were perceived to be momentous and requiring system change. However, most countries were nonetheless reluctant to embark on such major policy reform. Most preferred a slower, incremental approach to transform policy infrastructure step by step – choosing evolution rather than innovation. This underestimates the importance of completing the changes in time to gain the longevity dividend before the end of the population transition. Though national experiences can be shared, each country has to customize policy ideas for its own context, its culture, and the rate of the population transition, rather than identically copying policy ideas.

Japan is a 'super-aging society' with currently the highest proportion of older citizens of any country in the world. Japan can thus serve as a longevity laboratory for other countries, although some of its unique characteristics also must be considered. In 2021, persons aged 65 years and over accounted for 28.8% of the population (Cabinet Office, 2021). The share of the total population aged 75 years and over is larger (14.9%) than the share aged 65 to 74 (13.9). Due to this development, the Joint Committee of Japan Gerontological Society and the Japan Geriatrics Society proposed that the definition of elderly be changed to people aged 75 and over. Over 40% of those 65 and over would like to work in paid employment. The government projections suggest that one in 2.6 people will be aged 65 and over and one in 3.9 people will be aged 75 and over by 2065. Japan has over 80,000 centenarians, which will rise to 440,000 by 2050. In 2019, Japan's supercentenarians, or people aged 111 years and over, numbered 150. Many of them are women (D'Ambrogio, 2020). Above average life expectancy is not uncommon, sometimes described as 'age inflation', where people display characteristics of younger ages. Japan provides valuable experience, but its unique population structure suggests emulating cautiously. For instance, because of Japan's very low birth rate, the total population will decline rapidly, though the share of the population aged 65 years and over will continue to grow up to 38% in 2060. Japan undoubtedly provides some valuable policy ideas. It has pioneered new thinking about the value of the silver economy, long term care and 'agetech' technology.

Because of multiple policy interactions, planning for a whole-of-government response to population aging has been attempted in some countries. Holding public consultations, setting up expert or advisory committees or preparing reports or plans can be part of such efforts. The United Kingdom consulted experts for a foresight review and issued the report entitled 'Future of an Ageing Population' (Government Office for Science, 2016). Japan addressed the 100-year life society by establishing a dedicated council (Council for Designing 100-Year Life Society, 2017). It engaged experts and representatives of diverse disciplines and experience to generate policy ideas to facilitate the transition to a long-lived society. Japan's government reports annually on the implementation status of measures in six different domains – Employment and income; Health and welfare; Learning and social participation; Living environment; Research development and contribution to the world; and Promote success of all generations (Cabinet Office, 2021). Singapore launched its Action plan for successful aging, which included 70 initiatives and targets in twelve areas – health and wellness, learning, volunteerism, employment, housing, transport, public spaces, respect and social inclusion, retirement adequacy, healthcare and aged care, protection for vulnerable seniors and research (Ministry of Health, 2016). These countries exemplify steps to apply systemic thinking in order to adapt to longer life expectancy in their populations by simultaneously responding in many policy areas. Converting plans into result-producing actions is of course an additional challenge.

Compared to the 28.8% of older people in the population in Japan, the European Union average in 2019 was 20.5% (D'Ambrogio, 2020). The Scandinavian countries with high proportions of older people were early adopters of aging policies for housing and home care, and they continue to lead in supporting autonomy in later life. For instance, Denmark stopped building nursing homes, made collective homes more residential than institutional and implemented social services for aging at home as early as 1998 (Stuart and Weinrich, 2001). Preventive home visits postponed the need for more costly care. Countries can monitor the immediate and long-term impacts of these policies before emulating them.

7.2 Population Aging Determinism or Managed Policy Evolution?

The social policy infrastructure has been in place for decades in most countries. Policies for health, education, social support and pensions have well established histories. Many of them were developed at the time of the first population shift, when the birth rate was high but life expectancies were short. They have not faced the strains imposed by population aging. Will older cohorts be a burden on society, bankrupting public pensions and over-consuming expensive health services? Or will public policies be redesigned for a longer life span and handle each generation in the shifting population structure fairly? If the policy system does not evolve, population aging will be the major determinant of the societal outcomes of the population transition.

The evolution of policies for health, income security, economic and social participation and lifelong learning will have positive impacts on individuals and society. All citizens will have longer health spans, better income security, protected standards of living, access to current knowledge and skills and increased ability to contribute to society. Society will benefit from economic and social contributions from the whole adult population, economic and social growth and reduced public costs.

Strategic foresight has allowed some countries to make important choices and take actions that will benefit living and future generations living longer lives. Some of the policy experiences of countries and research evidence are captured below.

7.3 Policies for Lifelong Health, Longer Health Span and Active Living

7.3.1 Lifelong Health Care Culture

The health span is the number of years of life when a person is in general good physical and mental health. A longer health span increases the number of years of active living. It is well accepted that health in later years is built over the lifetime. This means that thinking in terms of medical treatments of the ailments associated with aging, e.g., replacement of joints, must shift to ensuring adequate access to health resources throughout life. Promoting health through life can be considered as a long-term investment with later returns in the form of lower acute care medical costs. Physical fitness and mental sharpness are built by health habits and health care practiced from childhood.

Aging varies among individuals in ways that are hidden in averages. Delaying age related conditions have huge benefits. Health promoting habits have helped people to stay healthy through most of their lives. In the United States, the increase in disability free life was greater than the increase in disabled life (Crimmins et al., 2016). With current medical practice even chronic or disabling conditions can be managed to enable an active and autonomous life.

7.3.2 Healthy Aging Improves Active Living and Societal Contributions

While a lifelong health policy that results in healthy aging likely raises health expenditure, the greater returns to society would partly or more than offset the increase. Good health while aging improves citizens' quality of life and their societal participation. There is a clear relationship between health expenditure and life expectancy where, in general, greater per capita expenditure is related to higher life expectancy. However, some countries are more efficient in gaining better outcomes for their public health expenditure. For example, among six countries that in 2019 had an average life expectancy of 83 years at birth, the per capita health costs varied widely. Norway spent US$ 8007, compared to US$ 6275 in Iceland, US$ 5427 in Australia, US$ 3456 in Israel, US$ 2625 in South Korea, and US$ 2532 in Malta

(World Bank, 2023). Japan and Singapore, with spending levels per capita at the lower end of this range, achieved somewhat longer life expectancy.

Biological evidence has demonstrated how aging has been dramatically changed by improving health throughout life. Improving the health of older people can increase the economic and social benefits that can be provided for the greater good. One estimate put the economic value of delayed aging over 50 years in the United States at around US$ 7 trillion (Goldman, 2016). The World Health Organization and European Observatory on Health Systems and Policies (2021) estimated how much a 5% decrease in disability rates through healthy aging among 55- to 69-year-olds would, cumulatively by the end of the century, contribute to additional growth in GDP per person. The estimates ranged from 31 percentage points in Mongolia to 55 percentage points in Korea, with Japan, Viet Nam, New Zealand, and Australia positioned in the middle or upper end of the range.

Good health pays off in rebalancing costs and benefits in later years of life. In countries that spend more on health promotion through the life course, more older people work, consume wisely, spend prudently and contribute to society through volunteering. People who are in good health are over four times more likely to work between the ages of 50 and 65 years rather than retiring early (Dimitriadis & Swain, 2020). They are ten times more likely to continue working between 65 and 74 years of age. An increase of 0.1% in preventive health spending in G20 countries was associated with a 9% increase in annual spending by people over 60 and 10 hours more of volunteer work for each person aged 65 and over.

7.3.3 Rebalancing Health Promotion, Prevention, Primary and Acute Care

Though people are living longer, health care tends to focus on providing primary care and acute care. Although preventive care delays aging-related conditions and prolongs life, it is neglected. One study recommended that G20 economies spend a minimum of 6% of health budgets on prevention (Dimitriadis & Swain, 2020). It also suggested that, after achieving that level, the target be raised to 15% of health budgets.

7.3.4 Supply and Distribution of Medical Specialists Should Keep Up with Changes in the Population

Geriatric medicine as a medical specialty is well established and contributes to greater longevity. However, the supply of geriatricians does not keep up with population aging in many countries. Basu et al. (2021) used a benchmark ratio of 1.25 specialists per 10,000 population over 65. By this measure, in Canada there was a widening estimated gap in the supply of geriatricians, with an estimated shortfall of 472 geriatricians in 2019. In many countries geriatricians tend to be located in large urban centres and hospitals, which makes equal geographical access to geriatric care an issue.

Managing the supply pipeline of specialists in step with population aging is a key means of ensuring that there are sufficient doctors for population health care. The present difference in the number of specialists can be stark. For example, in 2019, the Canadian Medical Association reported that there were 304 geriatricians and 2973 pediatricians in Canada, or 0.8 and 7.8, respectively, per 100,000 population (Basu et al., 2021).

Care at Home, Institutions or Hospitals and Pathways Across the System Based on the Needs of the Older Person at Specific Times

The health care needs of older persons can vary during later life, rather than increasing steadily. This means an older person may need intensive health care for a time and recover to good health and active living. A well-functioning system should have sufficient flexibility to allow people to move between residential arrangements depending on the care required at the time.

Long term care should be delivered in relation to need but also considering the preferences of the individual. Studies and polls show that older people overwhelmingly prefer to age at home. For example, in the United States, among people 50 to 80 years old, from 88 to 91% of respondents wanted to age in their own homes as long as possible (Pai, 2018; National Poll on Healthy Aging, 2022).

The idea that, with appropriate home care, more people can age in place at home is widely accepted. In Denmark, for example, Schulz (2010) reported that more older people lived at home with homecare services than lived in collective settings with care. Among those 85 to 89 years of age, three times as many persons received care at home as in institutional settings. Even among those 90 years and over, the number of persons living at home with home care was almost double the number living in institutional settings.

While reform often aims to shift occupancy from more expensive forms of care to those with lower costs, care should be appropriate to meet the needs. There should thus be pathways to move within the system, depending on temporary and growing needs and recognizing that not all people move through the system from lower to higher forms of care. If there is a co-pay requirement, it should be calibrated not to bankrupt older people or deprive them of the care needed for a decent quality of life.

7.3.5 *Recalibrating Public Costs of Health Care with Rates of Population Aging*

Long term care can be a mix of several types of care: hospital care, residential care, home care and informal care. With the demand for access to better quality care, this mix may change as part of health care reforms that could impact the costs of care. On average, 1.5% of GDP is allocated to long term care in OECD countries (OECD, 2020a). Countries that aged earlier, and started health care reform in response, spend more, which contributes to noticeable outcomes in health, quality of life and active living. The Netherlands, Denmark, Norway and Sweden spend around 3.5% of GDP for well-developed long term care systems. Switzerland, France, Belgium, Finland, United Kingdom, Germany and Japan allocate between 2% and 2.5% of GDP for long term care.

The rate of increase of expenditures on long term care depends not only on the growth of the aging population but also on the stage of long term care policy in the country and the composition of its types of care. The Netherlands historically had a generous program of long term care, spending 3.4% of GDP as early as 2005 (OECD, 2020c). It embarked on a process of reform, where financial responsibilities were transferred from the central authorities to the local level in 2015, and services were more oriented towards home care, which reduced the use of more expensive inpatient long term care. In contrast, in countries that are aging more slowly, such as Chile, Greece and Turkey, care has been provided by unpaid family members or paid by personal outlay. They are now beginning a process of planning for a more formal and comprehensive system.

The effectiveness of health care does not necessarily rely on high expenditure. Some countries have achieved greater life expectancy with lower health care spending per person than others. Access to and equity of care seem important, since the relationship between health expenditures and longevity is strongest in countries with an established public health care system. Such factors may help to explain the lower life expectancy seen in the United States than in other developed countries (Fig. 7.1).

7.3.6 *Potential Additional Supportive Costs*

Very few countries can manage without family or informal care. Spouses, mostly older women, provide unpaid care. Caring family members may be exposed to high stress and burnout, especially when caring for persons with major disabilities or dementia for long daily hours over extended periods of time. Until recently such care was unpaid. The value of this informal care and the carers' need for respite is sometimes recognized with financial compensation. In 2016, 15.9 million family members and friends in the United States provided 18.2 billion hours of unpaid care

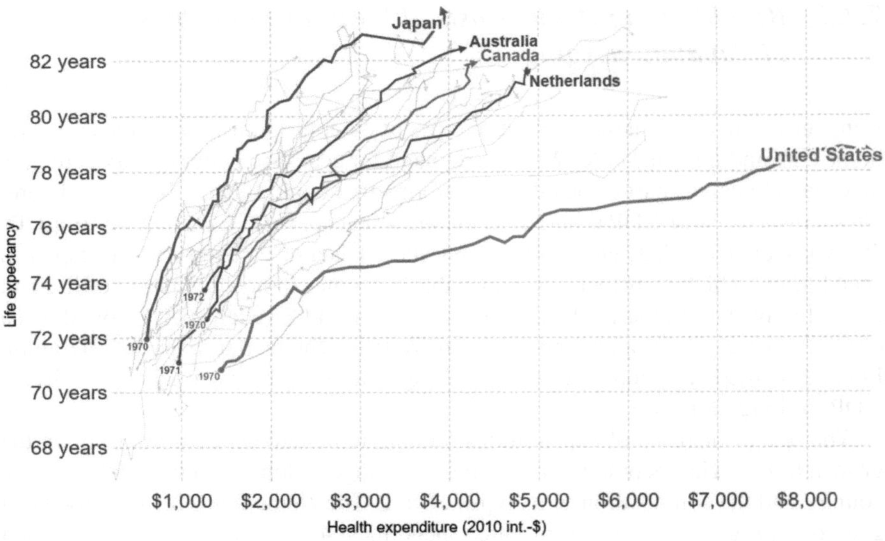

Fig. 7.1 Some countries have achieved greater life expectancy with lower health care spending per person than others. The relationship between health care spending per person and life expectancy in selected countries between 1970 and 2015. Selection of OECD data reproduced from Roser (2017). CC BY
Note: OECD data on total health expenditures financed by private and public sources. Health spending measures the consumption of health care goods and services, including personal health care (curative care, rehabilitation care, long-term care, ancillary services and medical goods) and collective services (prevention and public health services as well as health administration but excluding spending on investments)

to people with Alzheimer's and other dementias, worth an estimated US$ 230 billion worth of care (AgingWell Hub, 2018).

Supportive or 'cash for care' costs could add to the budgetary health expenditures, depending on the choice of policy. Israel and the Czech Republic pay the same benefits to formal as to informal carers. England pays cash benefits to the care recipients, while the Netherlands pays hourly wages to caregivers (Dyer et al., 2020).

Even when a person lives in assisted living, residential care or institutions, family and friends render a valuable service by maintaining family connections and providing social stimulation, security and exposure to culture and recreation. Many institutions depend on family members to feed their relative at meal times and to ensure that they are well hydrated.

7.4 Integration into the Economy

7.4.1 The Silver Economy

The economy in countries with a high proportion of older people benefits from the 'silver economy'. A part of the market system of production, distribution and consumption of goods and services is geared towards the purchasing potential of older people. Satisfying their needs for consumption, living and health is described as the silver economy. One estimate valued this consumer spending at more than US$ 8 trillion globally in 2020, rising to US$ 15 trillion in 2030 as population and incomes grow (Fengler, 2021). Since Western countries are richer and older than most other parts of the world, they account for the largest part of the global silver economy. The total annual spending power of older people is relatively equally distributed across Asia, Europe and North America (about US$ 2.3 trillion each). As the aging population grows in numbers in large economy countries, such as China and India, they will account for a larger share of the silver economy. By 2030, older people in Asia are expected to spend over US$ 5 trillion each year (Fengler, 2021).

Older consumers fuel the economy by their purchase of not only age-related goods but also goods and services from other sectors, such as mobile phones and hair salons. In 2015, spending by older households in G20 countries averaged 22% of GDP, amounting to almost USD 10 trillion, more than the GDP of many countries (Dimitriadis & Swain, 2020). However, they could spend more if they did not face barriers, such as products and services not being inclusive enough. Assuming that barriers to spending by people 75 years and over in the United Kingdom were removed by 2025, Dimitriadis (2019) estimated that by 2040 their spending could add 2% to GDP a year. If that age group could by 2025 match the spending of those 65–74, the addition to GDP by 2040 could be several times larger.

Policies for older consumers need a proactive perspective. With an increasing portion of consumer spending occurring on-line, older consumers could be helped to adapt to this development. New consumer goods may be of value to older consumers, but they may need more technological savvy to purchase them. With proper design, services such as home security or requests for home care or emergency services could be made accessible by simply pressing a button. High speed internet needs to be not only available but also affordable for all older consumers. As government services are shifting to digital provision, such as tax filing and passport renewals, affordable internet service is vital. St. Vincent and the Grenadines implemented subsidized access to the internet (Marius, 2021). The Canadian government in partnership with major telecommunications companies supports high speed internet for low-income older persons at a relatively low price (C$ 20 per month) through its Connecting Families initiative (Government of Canada, 2022).

Further innovation in products and services is to be expected. For example, among Americans aged 50 years and over, 18% were interested in driverless cars (AARP Research, 2021). They could help to solve transportation issues for consumers of advanced age, but targeted marketing initiatives might be needed to make such cars accessible to them.

7.4.2 Encouraging Personal Savings and Investments and Well Managed Public Pensions

Older cohorts have lived through wars and recessions, but they have also lived through periods of prosperity. Individuals have invested in their homes and they have been careful savers. They may be able to financially assist their children, donate to worthy causes and leave legacies. They are an important part of the economy through their property ownership and their investments, which are also transferred to the next generation through bequests.

In some developed countries, the size of assets in retirement savings plans is large enough to be more than double the size of the economy, such as 213% of GDP in the Netherlands in 2020 (OECD, 2021). Such plans in many other developed countries are large but with much less assets. Smaller amounts in public pension reserve funds, summing to almost US$ 7 trillion in OECD countries in 2020, complement the retirement savings plans (OECD, 2021). Public and private funds together can thus be a major source of funds for older people in many countries. Pension funds are some of the major world investors supporting the economy. The assets need to be governed and managed carefully in the face of economic vagaries so they can offer income security in old age.

7.4.3 Changes in Working Life and Participation in the Labour Market

Japan is a super aged country, meaning that more than one in five people in the country is 65 years or older. But in about a decade, Germany, France, the United Kingdom and Singapore (and others) will likely join Japan with this characteristic. These economic power houses will face a labour shortage if they do not have inclusive labour market policies.

Growing Share of Older Workers in the Labour Force

As the labour force shrinks, there is growing awareness of an untapped labour pool, consisting of older people with considerable knowledge, skills and experience. Compared to previous generations, more people aged over 65 have longer lives, better health and education, less high-risk working lives, and less physically demanding jobs or professions. The work world is finding it profitable to adapt and modify where, when and how work is done. Society gains from making better and longer use of this pool of knowledge and skills in the older population. Employers benefit from the retention of human capital, work experience and corporate memory. Attitudes of employers, workers and society are in the process of changing. The evidence that older people engage in paid work is growing. Promotion of employment of older workers contributed to the rise by an average of two and a half years in the effective age of labour market exit in OECD countries in a decade (OECD, 2019).

Some older individuals have to work to earn income for the years in retirement. While in 2018 the employment rate of persons in the 70 to 74 age group was 15% on average in OECD countries, it was 33% in Korea (OECD, 2020b). Korea also ranked highest among OECD countries with a 44% share of people over 65 years who were in relative poverty (less than half of the median income).

In the United States, in the decade of 2014–2024, the annual growth rates in the labour force of the age groups 65–74 years and 75 years and over were estimated to be, respectively, 55% and 86% (Toossi & Torpey, 2017). The corresponding rate for the labour force as a whole would be 5%. In 2024, the age group 65 and over would then constitute about 8% of the labour force. While in G20 countries the employment rate of people aged 50 to 69 was 57% in 2017, it could rise to 65% in 2035, which would be close to the rate of younger adults (Dimitriadis & Swain, 2020).

Policies that encourage retaining older workers in the labour market operate in several countries. In the United States, for example, the Age Discrimination in Employment Act of 1967 was enacted already that early to prohibit such discrimination (specific provisions subsequently updated through amendments). International provisions and protections regarding labour and social issues are stipulated in conventions and recommendations of the United Nations International Labour Organization. In particular, the Older Workers Recommendation, 1980 (No. 162) deals with equality of opportunity, fair treatment and access to employment-related services, such as counselling (Samorodov, 1999).

In many countries, people are also eager to continue working beyond age 65 for satisfaction and social interaction. Some have switched to second or 'encore' careers. Others choose to work part-time, short-term or as advisors and mentors. A few become investors and entrepreneurs in business ventures.

Working Longer Results in Substantial Gains to GDP

The projected labour shortage is stimulating supply and demand policies that are more inclusive. More job flexibility is possible because much work can be done remotely, part-time or even as self-employment. Halvorsen (2021) points out that the employment rates of older workers in the Nordic countries are particularly high and also rising, based on OECD data. The employment rates in Iceland in 2019 demonstrate what can be achieved: 78%, 50% and 15%, respectively, in the age groups 60–64 years, 65–69 years and 70–74 years. Dimitriadis and Swain (2020) projected that if older workers in G20 economies in 2035 were employed at the same rates as in Iceland, these economies could anticipate an average GDP gain of 7% (about US$ 3.7 trillion).

Growth in the employment rate of workers aged over 65 is possible in most countries. The skills and work experience of involuntarily unemployed older workers can fill skill shortages and increase process innovation. Workers aged 50 and over earned every third dollar in the G20 economies in 2014, which could rise to nearly 40% by 2035 (Dimitriadis & Swain, 2020).

Removing Mandatory Retirement

The hard boundary between work and retirement is disappearing. The attraction of 'freedom 55' early retirement of the 1980s is waning. Several OECD countries no longer allow employers to set a mandatory retirement age (Australia, Canada, Denmark, New Zealand, Poland, United Kingdom, United States), although this is still possible in many other countries (OECD, 2017a). Many countries wish to retain a more flexible eligibility for policies based on age. In addition, incentives to delay retirement and removal of disincentives attached to pensions encourage retention in the workforce.

7.5 Raising the Pension Age

Future effective retirement pension ages will continue to rise. Assuming labour market entry in 2020 at the age of 22 years, the normal retirement age will increase to 66.1 for men and 65.5 for women on average across all OECD countries (OECD, 2021). This is an increase of some 2 years from 2020. Higher retirement age will also follow when countries increase the age of eligibility for public retirement programs to above age 65, which numerous countries have either done or are in the process of doing. A higher pension eligibility age needs to be complemented with income support for those older people who are unable to work.

7.5.1 Linking the Age of Retirement to Life Expectancy

An alternative to a fixed age for pension eligibility is to link the statutory age of retirement to life expectancy. In other words, the age of retirement and pension eligibility is based on prospective age (or years of life remaining), which reduces the years in retirement progressively with increasing life expectancy. Whitehouse (2007) identified thirteen countries with a link between pensions and life expectancy (Australia, Denmark, Finland, France, Germany, Hungary, Italy, Mexico, Norway, Poland, Portugal, Slovakia, Sweden). Five countries (Denmark, Finland, Italy, the Netherlands, and Portugal) will index the age of eligibility for their primary pension programs to life expectancy (Eisen et al., 2022). The retirement age will thus automatically adjust upward as life expectancy grows. It is anticipated that this will both increase the pension savings of individuals and ensure the sustainability of pension systems (OECD, 2019).

7.5.2 Flexible Retirement and Phased Retirement Options

Bridging the transition to retirement or phased retirement can encourage older workers to work less but longer. Pension policies can allow a combination of work and pension income without penalty. In Sweden, some municipalities and regional governments offer their public sector workers an 80–90-100 model of phased retirement for 3 years at age 62. The worker can work 80% of time for 90% of the pay and full contribution to his or her pension plan (Wahlstein, 2023).

Because of longer life expectancy, people can live in retirement for 25 years or more. Despite working longer, both men and women can still expect to spend between one-fifth and a quarter of their lives, or even more, in retirement. The introduction of options to ensure adequate pension income in retirement has been beneficial, but not all people can take advantage of these schemes (OECD, 2019). For instance, the swing to defined contribution pension schemes has had a negative effect on low income people by shifting the risk to them.

Longer working years benefit workers, employers and public programs. Retirees are more likely to work if they are highly educated, live in urban areas or have a mortgage. The introduction of policies for flexible retirement options and for delayed retirement reduces the likelihood of a savings gap for the non-working years (OECD, 2019). Flexible retirement policies aim to foster the combination of work and pensions as a gradual withdrawal from the labour market. The simplest form of combining work and pensions is to claim a full pension at the normal retirement age and to continue working part-time or full-time beyond this age. No OECD country requires workers to stop working entirely at the normal retirement age. However, some countries limit how much pensioners can earn, which can be a deterrent. In some countries, deferring pensions pays a pension bonus of 6 to 8% for each year of deferral, in addition to the higher entitlements earned when working (OECD, 2017a). Such provisions are seen in, for example, Canada, Denmark, Japan and the United Kingdom. The bonus can be partially offset if other benefits subject to income-testing are withdrawn, as can be the case in Canada and Denmark.

7.5.3 Financial Incentives

To make it worthwhile for older workers to work longer, the removal of tax and other disincentives and penalties for earned income in retirement can be considered. Complementary tax-free retirement savings programs can further supplement pension income (OECD, 2019).

7.6 Intergenerational Exchanges and Transfers

During the evolution of humans as social beings, parents invested heavily in their children through many years of dependency. This behavior morphed into other forms of transfers, even after children had grown. Transfers are donations between generations without expectation of repayment. Intergenerational transfers are often misconstrued as solely wealth or economic transfers within families. However, they also include transfers from one generation to the other of non-economic resources valuable for life. Various forms of care, emotional support, and promotion of education are examples of such transfers, as is the access for the younger generation to social networks that can provide a leg up in their start to independent life. It is a means of reallocating advantage from one generation to the other and to promote upward social mobility and social progress. Care of the older generation by the younger is an indication of reciprocal exchanges over time.

7.6.1 Unpaid Work, Volunteering and Care Giving by Older Citizens

The rate of employment declines significantly after age 65. People in this older age group are nevertheless, even if not involved in paid employment, a major proportion of the voluntary sector. They contribute care, expertise, money and time. Dimitriadis and Swain (2020) found that the average unpaid contributions of older people in the European Union and Turkey could be worth as much as 1.4% of GDP. The value of older people's non-market contributions is greater than often assumed, exceeding the expenditure on defence in some countries, for example.

7.6.2 Work in the Caring Economy

The contributions made by the older population in care giving are vastly underestimated. Colombo et al. (2011) recognized that in most countries family carers and friends supply the majority of care, and its estimated economic value exceeds by far the expenditures on formal care. Public budgets and infrastructure would not be able to care for the old, demented, ill and disabled citizens without the informal care giving provided by family members, sometimes by spouses who are aging themselves. Governments have only in recent decades begun supporting such caregivers. This can take the form of policies for leave with or without pay, flexible work, tax credits and allowances, training and respite care.

7.6.3 Contributions Associated with Roles and Functions of Older People in Family Life

The processes that change how populations are composed also cause changes to family structures. Greater longevity means that, previously rare, four or even five generations could be alive in the family. For the first time, families comprise more adults than children. These changes have an impact on family functions and traditional exchanges between family members. Taking a life-course perspective allows societies to support families and children through the life span.

Older members of the family are in better health than in earlier times. They can therefore not only care for themselves but also provide care for other members of the family. Grandparenting has grown in importance, particularly when both of the children's parents work. As the youth generation spends more time in education, they may live in the family home for longer periods of time and have more contact with the older generations.

Older family members may have invested in property and savings, which can strengthen financial security both for themselves and for younger generations in the family. Legacies from older members may transfer assets to younger family members. Older generations may assist with the educational costs of younger generations or help with down-payments for the purchase of housing.

Transfers and bequests can be not only financial in nature but also intangible. The older people link families to previous generations. They can explain family health history through inherited genes, demonstrate family recipes, and share tacit knowledge or know-how and tricks of the family trade. They remember family networks, family traditions and celebrations. Anthropologists and gerontologists are creating methodologies to preserve this legacy.

7.7 Lifelong Learning

The relationship between healthy aging and lifelong learning is synergistic, providing a combined value greater than their individual impacts. The societal benefits of the longevity dividend are much higher when lifelong learning continues through a healthy later life. Lifelong learning, like life itself, is longitudinal, cumulative and holistic. Initial learning increases literacy, learning skills and work-related knowledge. Subsequent learning through the rest of life improves health and active living and also supports the learning of new skills and updating knowledge while aging in a transforming world. The benefits of lifelong learning flow to the individual and to society.

Individuals embedded in a learning culture consider the constant acquisition of knowledge and skills a life activity. Knowledge is the best safety net for an individual's autonomy and health, especially if it is a part of the rhythm of daily activities. Lifelong learning improves the quality of life for individuals by enabling better self-care and life management, informed management of risk and opportunities and prudent decision making in matters of a health, financial and legal nature. Lifelong learning affects the effectiveness, adaptability and fulfillment of individuals in life as well as their success in society. It expands career options, sustains personal growth and facilitates achieving one's personal best in life.

With lifelong learning the contributions individuals make to society are more effective because they are based on individuals having made accurate appraisals of need, chosen best options and applied the latest knowledge and skills. Lifelong learning supplies the evidence for individual decisions and collective societal choices for the current and future generations. The wiser choices made by society celebrate the long and growing life expectancy of individuals by valuing the contributions they made in various roles during the entirety of life.

Lifelong learning ensures that the individual and societal stocks of knowledge and skills are retained, and increased with evolving knowledge, so they can be applied to the enhancement of social progress. Furthermore, lifelong learning helps to make the later years worthwhile for individuals and society by capitalizing on the gains from the longevity dividend. These gains are immediate and also extend into the future.

7.8 Policies for Lifelong Learning

Lifelong learning by individuals is voluntary, but not engaging in lifelong learning can impose low returns all through life or unavoidable losses in wellbeing. People with higher levels of education tend to engage in more education and lifelong learning (OECD, 2017b). This can impel a virtuous cycle of benefits for society. On the other hand, inequalities in education, health, and employment magnify over time, resulting in large differences in lifetime outcomes which create social inequities. Poorly distributed lifelong learning can result in unequal opportunities for citizens and higher public costs.

The need to prevent inter- and intra-generation inequities and the promise of higher benefits from the longevity dividend have encouraged both international organizations of governments and national governments to develop policy action for increased learning. Governments that take the opportunity to extend their education infrastructure to include people in later life will gain both short- and long-term benefits.

7.9 International Policy Initiatives for Lifelong Learning

International organizations have been involved in the democratization of knowledge and lifelong learning for decades. To play an active role in encouraging lifelong learning, they rely on 'soft power', research and communication because public policies are the responsibility of national governments. But their contributions are essential for informing national governments and supporting them in promoting progress and reducing inequities. While international organizations of member governments have launched many initiatives, they rarely, if at all, specifically promote later life learning as the last stage in lifelong learning. The idea may nonetheless be implicit in their initiatives.

The following selective inventory highlights a number of international and national policy initiatives for lifelong learning.

7.9.1 World Bank

The titles of these two initiatives convey succinctly their key dimensions: Lifelong learning in the global knowledge economy (World Bank, 2003) and Ending learning poverty and building skills (World Bank, 2021).

7.9.2 United Nations

Multiple organizations in the United Nations system have established a regular process for monitoring and producing important work that will guide their member nations in making policy decisions.

The UNESCO Convention against Discrimination in Education was adopted in 1960. It is a legally binding international instrument entirely dedicated to the right to education. Signatories are held responsible for violations of the right to education. National reports are monitored.

The United Nations Economic and Social Council [ECOSOC] has promoted four interrelated criteria for judging the implementation of rights to education. These are availability, accessibility, acceptability and adaptability to societal context (Tomaševski, 2001).

The United Nations Sustainable Development Agenda was adopted in 2015 with a 2030 deadline for reaching its 17 goals. These Sustainable Development Goals to be achieved by 2030 are a call for action by all countries to promote prosperity, while protecting the planet and ensuring all people enjoy peace and prosperity. The Sustainable Developmental Goal 4 specifically addresses lifelong learning. It aims to ensure inclusive and equitable quality education and promote lifelong learning opportunities for all (United Nations, 2015).

7.9.3 UNESCO Institute for Lifelong Learning (UIL)

Embracing a culture of lifelong learning (UIL, 2020) is UIL's contribution to the UNESCO International Commission on the Futures of Education. It promotes the creation of a global culture of lifelong learning in order to address the challenges faced by humanity, whether it is climate change or technological disruptions.

7.9.4 European Parliament

The European Parliament adopted a resolution during its eighth term (2014–2019), stating that education is a fundamental right and a public good that should be adequately resourced and be equally accessible to all (European Parliamentary Research Service, n.d.). In the resolution adopted in the ninth term (2019–2024), the Parliament reiterated its support for inclusivity.

The European Parliament, the Council and the European Commission proclaimed the *European Pillar of Social Rights* in 2017. Among its 20 principles, the first principle is Education, training and lifelong learning. It states that everyone has the right to quality and inclusive education, training and lifelong learning in order to maintain and acquire skills that enable them to participate fully in society and to successfully manage transitions in the labour market (European Commission, 2021).

7.9.5 European Commission

The European area of lifelong learning aims to empower citizens to move freely between learning settings, jobs, regions and countries, and to be more inclusive, tolerant and democratic (European Commission, 2001). It enables them to make the most of their knowledge and competencies to meet the goals and ambitions of the European Union.

7.9.6 Organization for Economic Cooperation and Development (OECD)

In 1996, the education ministers in OECD countries adopted 'Lifelong learning for all' as a policy framework. The organization summarized its work over the subsequent 5 years in a document dedicated to lifelong learning for all, including analysis of policy directions and stocktaking (OECD, 2001).

7.10 Current National Policy Approaches for Lifelong Learning

Societal learning is valuable in order to learn from the experimentation in peer countries. Achieving transformative change for lifelong learning can be a difficult task, particularly in terms of integrating established systems of education into a larger lifelong system. Longstanding ministries can have names that reveal their priorities, such as early childhood education, or compulsory schooling and higher education, in contrast to the lifelong perspective. As attempts are being made to introduce a lifelong learning priority, congruence in policy intent may be achievable while policy implementation lags behind. Lifelong learning cannot be an auxiliary system but is rather an overarching governing framework for all types of learning.

The most widely used strategy is for a country to define the concept of lifelong learning and to describe the rationale for implementing it through policy, citing potential national and citizen benefits. Since this strategy only signals the desired national policy direction, individuals and families have to make deliberate decisions. Such policy implementation relies on 'exhortation' or persuasion rather than coercion (Doern & Wilson, 1974).

The documentation centre and library of the UNESCO Institute for Lifelong Learning (UIL) contains policy documents on Lifelong Learning Policies and Strategies collected from UNESCO members, which forms a valuable resource (UIL, 2023). Forty-three countries have some policy or strategy for lifelong learning, as surveyed by the UIL in 2023. Countries often described their concept of lifelong learning using terms such as 'cradle to grave' or 'life span' in the description in order to set it apart from life stage education. Some pointed out that it was everyone's shared responsibility. The rationale included the benefits to both individuals and the country. Countries had ambitious goals. Denmark aims to help 'future-proof Denmark'. Finland stated that a challenge was to raise the level of education among the population as a whole and constantly develop the national knowledge reserve. Kenya had a Vision 2030, noting that it is necessary to empower individuals to become self-determined and educated citizens through lifelong learning.

Some countries took a long-term comprehensive approach to provide a systemic view of education with national objectives. Consider the example of Estonia

(European Commission, 2022). Estonia had made several earlier unsuccessful attempts to create an encompassing strategy for lifelong learning. Starting in 2014, the European Union required a national policy framework for lifelong learning for the granting of structural funds. This energized the process where the Estonian Cooperation Assembly, the Estonian Education Forum and the Ministry of Education and Research worked together to draft a strategy through wide public consultations. The measures and activities of the strategy were approved by the country's parliament in 2014. On this foundation, the Estonian Lifelong Learning Strategy 2021–2035 was developed with the overall objective to equip the people of Estonia with the knowledge, skills and attitudes to fulfil their potential in personal, occupation and social life, while simultaneously promoting the quality of life in Estonia and contributing to global sustainable development. The three strategic goals to achieve this objective were (1) to provide diverse and accessible learning opportunities in an education system that enables smooth transitions between levels and types of education, (2) to develop a corps of competent and motivated teachers and heads of learning institutions that rely on a learner-centred approach to learning while teaching in diverse learning environments and (3) to offer learning options that are responsive to the development needs of the labour market and society. The implementation of the strategy would be monitored using predetermined indicators.

Other countries have resorted to a shorter term and incremental approach, announcing an umbrella policy or legislation or setting up a cabinet committee for lifelong learning to incorporate existing components. This makes it difficult to determine any particular policy actions on lifelong learning taken under legislative initiatives. The approach nevertheless adds value by taking a systemic view of education with connections and continuity between components.

Several countries, including Japan, Korea, Norway, Thailand and the United States, have passed a 'Lifelong Learning Act' (UIL, 2023). As early as 1976, the United States made amendments to the Higher Education Act to include lifelong learning, often popularly referred to as the Lifelong Learning Act (Education Amendments of 1976, 1976).

Some common themes pursued in countries' legislation related to lifelong learning have been as follows.

- Increase learning by citizens throughout life: The document for the lifelong learning strategy of Scotland is entitled: Life Through Learning Through Life (Scottish Executive, 2003).
- Increase the learning opportunities equitably among citizens: The act in the United States aims to increase lifelong learning opportunities without restrictions from previous education and training, sex, age, handicapping conditions, social and ethnic background and economic circumstances (Education Amendments of 1976, 1976).
- Increase the stock of human capital: The Scottish Strategy for lifelong learning states that the benefits of learned knowledge and skills are for individuals to improve their position in the labour market and increase productivity and

earnings which would collectively enhance the society in which they live (Scottish Executive, 2003).

7.10.1 Government Ministers or Departments

Some countries have named Cabinet Secretaries or Ministers of Lifelong Learning, often in combination with another portfolio. However, there appears to be some lack of permanence. To implement policies, a few governments have set up a department or a bureau of lifelong learning. Some examples include the following.

Scotland. The position of Minister for Enterprise and Lifelong Learning was created in 1999 in Scotland (Minister for Enterprise and Lifelong Learning, 2023). The role was changed to Minister for Enterprise, Transport and Lifelong Learning in 2002. In 2009, the Cabinet secretary for Education and Lifelong Learning was appointed. The post no longer exists.

Canada. The Province of Prince Edward Island named a Minister for Education and Lifelong Learning in 2021 (Department of Education and Lifelong Learning, 2023).

Japan. MEXT, the Ministry of Education in Japan, had a Lifelong Learning Policy Bureau (UIL, 2008).

7.11 National Lifelong Learning Policies that Specifically Include People in their Later Years

Some countries have reported that they had policies planned for people in later life. A few examples follow.

7.11.1 Austria: Strategy for Lifelong Learning, Lifelong Learning 2020 Issued in 2011

The Austrian Strategy for Lifelong Learning will invest in existing learning infrastructure to include and promote learning opportunities for retired persons (UIL, 2011). Guidance counselling and information on educational opportunities will be provided to increase their participation. Educators working with older learners are expected to obtain competencies relevant for teaching them and to use innovative pedagogic models to maintain quality. Where possible, learning opportunities will be provided close to their homes while taking into account intergenerational and technology enhanced learning. The strategy will also intensify research to improve learning opportunities for this group.

7.11.2 Finland: Ministry of Education Strategy 2015, Issued in 2003

The report The Joy of Learning, produced by a government committee, presented a national vision of lifelong learning (Ministry of Education, 1997). It aimed to promote intellectual growth through opportunities for comprehensive learning and self-development. Flexibility in the education system would recognize the results of informal learning. Lifelong learning would be used to promote the wellbeing of the aging population. Since its appearance, the report was updated in 2003 and 2015. The multiple goals of lifelong learning were confirmed through public consultations. The document was accepted by the Finnish Pension Alliance and a couple of pension insurance companies. It suggests that lifelong learning is about more than competencies, competitiveness and well-being. It is also the means to achieve education, inclusion and prevention of social inequality in society.

Sitra, an independent public foundation and think tank, reports directly to the Finnish parliament. Working with government and non-government stakeholders such as ministries, employers, unions and professional associations, it published a comparison of lifelong learning governance in the Nordic countries in 2021 (Ranki et al., 2021).

7.11.3 Japan: The Lifelong Learning Promotion Law, 1999

Japan was concerned about its 'hyper aging society' and the need for the aging population to be included in productive activities for wellbeing. The objective of the Strategy for lifelong learning was to create an enriching and dynamic society in the twenty-first century (Centre for Public Impact, 2018). This included a lifelong learning society. People would freely choose learning opportunities at any time during their lives, resulting in recognition of their learning achievements. The goals were to move beyond formal education and the 'diploma society' and to promote learning at all stages of life. The Ministry of Education allocated 8.5% of its 2007 budget to lifelong learning, which supported the creation of Lifelong Learning Councils at prefectural levels, surveys of people's learning needs and promotion of lifelong learning at the community level. Learning activities included sports, culture, hobbies, recreation and volunteer activities throughout civil society, universities and traditional community centres.

7.12 The Longevity Dividend Will Be Larger for Countries that Embrace the Challenges of Transformation

The perspective of the longevity dividend frames the aging of the population as an opportunity to achieve progress through creating value from the population shift (Jarvis, 2008). However, the policy responses require a lifelong perspective in which benefits accrue to all living generations.

The two strategies to enlarge the longevity dividend are, first, to implement policies which will increase the total productive contributions to society over the lifetime and, second to invest in lifelong learning in order to add greater societal value by improving the quality of these increased contributions. These strategies for enriching the longevity dividend are challenging for several reasons. The way forward requires a mental shift from seeing population aging as negative to seizing the opportunities it offers. Both strategies require 'creative disruption' (Dru, 1997) of the well-established policy structures for health, education and the economy. This means moving away from a focus on dependency ratios and labour market concerns about a burdened shrinking workforce. Policies have to be reframed to include a lifelong view and incorporate benefits to all ages. Because the potential for large gains from the longevity dividend is time limited, policy changes have to occur fairly quickly and simultaneously. The transformation needs to be accompanied by a culture change, which values population aging, respects the process of aging and endorses the role that older people play in society. The most demanding task is to develop a lifelong learning system that focusses on learning for citizens of all ages and which continually adapts to a changing context.

References

AARP Research. (2021). *2022 tech trends and the 50-plus* (Report). https://www.aarp.org/content/dam/aarp/research/surveys_statistics/technology/2021/2022-technology-trends-older-americans.doi.10.26419-2Fres.00493.001.pdf

AgingWell Hub. (2018). Resources and insights. *Georgetown University*. https://agingwellhub.org/resources-and-insights/

Basu, M., Cooper, T., Kay, K., Hogan, D. B., Morais, J. A., Molnar, F., Lam, R. E., & Borrie, M. J. (2021). Updated inventory and projected requirements for specialist physicians in geriatrics. *Canadian Geriatrics Journal, 24*(3), 200–208. https://doi.org/10.5770/cgj.24.538

Cabinet Office. (2021). *Annual report on the ageing society [summary] FY2021*. Government of Japan. https://www8.cao.go.jp/kourei/english/annualreport/index-wh.html

Centre for Public Impact. (2018, August 3). *Japan's lifelong learning promotion law*. https://www.centreforpublicimpact.org/case-study/lifelong-learning-japan

Colombo, F., Llena-Nozal, A., Mercier, J., & Tjadens, F. (2011). *Help wanted? Providing and paying for long-term care* (OECD Health Policy Studies). OECD Publishing. https://doi.org/10.1787/9789264097759-en

Council for Designing 100-Year Life Society. (2017, September 11). *The prime minister in action*. https://japan.kantei.go.jp/97_abe/actions/201709/11article5.html

Crimmins, E. M., Zhang, Y., & Saito, Y. (2016). Trends over 4 decades in disability-free life expectancy in the United States. *American Journal of Public Health, 106*(7), 1287–1293. https://doi.org/10.2105/AJPH.2016.303120

D'Ambrogio, E. (2020, December). *Japan's ageing society* (PE 659.419). European Parliamentary Research Service. https://www.europarl.europa.eu/RegData/etudes/BRIE/2020/659419/EPRS_BRI(2020)659419_EN.pdf

Department of Education and Lifelong Learning. (2023). *Education and lifelong learning*. Government of Prince Edward Island. https://www.princeedwardisland.ca/en/topic/education-and-lifelong-learning

Dimitriadis, S. (2019). *Maximising the longevity dividend.* International Longevity Centre UK. https://ilcuk.org.uk/wp-content/uploads/2019/12/Maximising-the-longevity-dividend.pdf

Dimitriadis, S., & Swain, P. (2020). *Health equals wealth: The global longevity dividend (report).* International Longevity Centre UK. https://ilcuk.org.uk/HealthEqualsWealth/

Doern, G. B., & Wilson, V. S. (Eds.). (1974). *Issues in Canadian public policy*. Macmillan.

Dru, J.-M. (1997). *Disruption: Overturning conventions and shaking up the marketplace*. Wiley.

Dyer, S. M., Valeri, M., Arora, N., Ross, T., Winsall, M., Tilden, D., & Crotty, M. (2020). *Review of international systems for long-term care of older people* (Research paper 2). Prepared for the Royal Commission into Aged Care Quality and Safety. https://agedcare.royalcommission.gov.au/publications/research-paper-2-review-international-systems-long-term-care-older-people

Education Amendments of 1976, Pub. L. No. 94–482 90 Stat. (1976). *United States 20 U.S.C.* https://www.govinfo.gov/content/pkg/STATUTE-90/pdf/STATUTE-90-Pg2081.pdf

Eisen, B., Lafleur, S., & Clemens, J. (2022). *The age of eligibility for public retirement programs in the OECD: 2022 update* (Research Bulletin). Fraser Institute. https://www.fraserinstitute.org/sites/default/files/age-of-eligibillity-for-public-retirement-programs-in-OECD-2022.pdf

European Commission. (2001, November 21). *Making a European area of lifelong learning a reality* (COM(2001) 678 final). Communication from the Commission. https://eur-lex.europa.eu/LexUriServ/LexUriServ.do?uri=COM:2001:0678:FIN:EN:PDF

European Commission. (2021). *The European pillar of social rights action plan.* https://op.europa.eu/webpub/empl/european-pillar-of-social-rights/downloads/KE0921008ENN.pdf

European Commission. (2022, October 19). *2.2 lifelong learning strategy.* Eurydice. Estonia. https://eurydice.eacea.ec.europa.eu/national-education-systems/estonia/lifelong-learning-strategy

European Parliamentary Research Service. (n.d.). *Lifelong learning in the EU.* https://www.europarl.europa.eu/thinktank/infographics/lifelonglearning/

Scottish Executive. (2003). *Life through learning through life: The lifelong learning strategy for Scotland.* https://dera.ioe.ac.uk//8815/

Fengler, W. (2021, January 14). The silver economy is coming of age: A look at the growing spending power of seniors. Brookings, Future Development. https://www.brookings.edu/blog/future-development/2021/01/14/the-silver-economy-is-coming-of-age-a-look-at-the-growing-spending-power-of-seniors/

Goldman, D. (2016). The economic promise of delayed aging. *Cold Spring Harbor Perspectives in Medicine, 18*(6), a025072. http://perspectivesinmedicine.cshlp.org/content/early/2015/12/18/cshperspect.a025072

Government of Canada. (2022, April 4). *Government of Canada announces affordable high-speed internet to help connect low-income families and seniors* [News release]. https://www.canada.ca/en/innovation-science-economic-development/news/2022/04/government-of-canada-announces-affordable-high-speed-internet-to-help-connect-low-income-families-and-seniors.html

Government Office for Science. (2016). *Future of an ageing population.* United Kingdom. https://assets.publishing.service.gov.uk/government/uploads/system/uploads/attachment_data/file/816458/future-of-an-ageing-population.pdf

Halvorsen, B. E. (2021). High and rising senior employment in the Nordic countries. *European Journal of Workplace Innovation., 6*(1–2), 130–146. https://pdfs.semanticscholar.org/ad18/265886f95e7a34581d46ecdf2efe39c80360.pdf?_ga=2.112620737.495617294.1626293667-1888582868.1626293667

Jarvis, P. (2008). *Democracy, lifelong learning and the learning society: Active citizenship in a late modern age*. Routledge.

Marius, M. (2021, March 19). Subsidized internet: What can we learn from countries that offer this programme? *ICT Pulse*. https://www.ict-pulse.com/2021/03/subsidized-internet-what-can-we-learn-from-countries-that-offer-that-programme/

Minister for Enterprise and Lifelong Learning. (2023, March 1). *In Wikipedia*. https://en.wikipedia.org/wiki/Minister_for_Enterprise_and_Lifelong_Learning

Ministry of Education. (1997). *The joy of learning: A national strategy for lifelong learning*. Report of the Committee for Lifelong Learning.

Ministry of Health. (2016). I feel young in my Singapore! In *Action plan for successful ageing*. Ministerial Committee on Ageing. https://sustainabledevelopment.un.org/content/documents/1525Action_Plan_for_Successful_Aging.pdf

National Poll on Healthy Aging. (2022). *Older adults' preparedness to age in place*. University of Michigan, Institute for Healthcare Policy and Innovation. https://doi.org/10.7302/4278

OECD. (2001). Education policy analysis 2001. In *Centre for educational research and innovation*. OECD Publishing. https://www.oecd-ilibrary.org/education/education-policy-analysis-2001_epa-2001-en

OECD. (2017a). *Pensions at a glance 2017*. OECD Publishing. https://doi.org/10.1787/19991363

OECD. (2017b). *Preventing ageing unequally*. OECD Publishing. https://doi.org/10.1787/9789264279087-en

OECD. (2019). *Working better with age: Ageing and employment policies*. OECD Publishing. https://doi.org/10.1787/c4d4f66a-en

OECD. (2020a). *Long-term care resources and utilization: Long-term care recipients*. OECD.Stat. Retrieved 30 January 2023. https://stats.oecd.org/index.aspx?queryid=30143

OECD. (2020b). *OECD economic surveys: Korea 2020*. OECD Publishing. https://doi.org/10.1787/2dde9480-en

OECD. (2020c, November). *Spending on long term care*. https://www.oecd.org/health/health-systems/Spending-on-long-term-care-Brief-November-2020.pdf

OECD. (2021). *Pensions at a glance 2021: OECD and G20 indicators*. OECD Publishing. https://www.oecd.org/publications/oecd-pensions-at-a-glance-19991363.htm

Pai, S. (2018). The rise of the silver economy. In *Georgetown Business* (Spring 2018), Georgetown University, McDonough School of Business. University. https://msb.georgetown.edu/news/georgetown-business-magazine/archive/.

Ranki, S., Ryky, P., Santamäki, I., & Smidt, H. (2021, January). *Lifelong learning governance in the Nordic countries: A comparison* (Memorandum). Sitra. https://www.sitra.fi/app/uploads/2021/01/lifelong-learning-governance-in-the-nordic-countries-1.pdf

Roser, M. (2017). *Link between health spending and life expectancy: The US is an outlier*. OurWorldInData.org [Based on data from OECD]. https://ourworldindata.org/the-link-between-life-expectancy-and-health-spending-us-focus

Samorodov, A. (1999). *Ageing and labour markets for older workers*. Employment and training papers 33. International Labour Organization. https://www.ilo.org/wcmsp5/groups/public/%2D%2D-ed_emp/documents/publication/wcms_120333.pdf

Schulz, E. (2010, May). *The long-term care system in Denmark* (ENEPRI Research Report No.73). European Network of Economic Policy Research Institutes. https://www.ceps.eu/ceps-publications/long-term-care-system-elderly-denmark/

Stuart, M., & Weinrich, M. (2001). Home- and community-based long-term care: Lessons from Denmark. *The Gerontologist, 41*(4), 474–480. https://doi.org/10.1093/geront/41.4.474

Tomaševski, K. (2001). *Human rights obligations: Making education available, accessible, acceptable and adaptable* (right to education primers no. 3). Right to education initiative. https://www.right-to-education.org/sites/right-to-education.org/files/resource-attachments/Tomasevski_Primer%203.pdf

Toossi, M., & Torpey, E. (2017, May). *Older workers: Labour force trends and career options.* United States Bureau of Labor Statistics, Career Outlook. https://www.bls.gov/careeroutlook/2017/article/older-workers.html

UNESCO Institute for Lifelong Learning. (2008). *Lifelong learning policy Bureau, ministry of education, culture, sports, science and technology (MEXT).* (Japan). https://uil.unesco.org/partner/lifelong-learning/lifelong-learning-policy-bureau-ministry-education-culture-sports-science

UNESCO Institute for Lifelong Learning. (2011). *Austria: Strategy for lifelong learning LLL:2020 issued in 2011.* https://uil.unesco.org/document/austria-strategy-lifelong-learning-lll2020-issued-2011

UNESCO Institute for Lifelong Learning. (2020). *Embracing a culture of lifelong learning: Contribution to the futures of education initiative.* https://uil.unesco.org/lifelong-learning/embracing-culture-lifelong-learning

UNESCO Institute for Lifelong Learning. (2023). *Collection of lifelong learning policies and strategies.* https://uil.unesco.org/lifelong-learning/lifelong-learning-policies

United Nations. (2015). *Transforming our world: The 2030 agenda for sustainable development. Resolution adopted by the general assembly on 25 September 2015* (A/RES/70/1). https://www.un.org/en/development/desa/population/migration/generalassembly/docs/globalcompact/A_RES_70_1_E.pdf

Wahlstein, I. (2023, March 3) *Vem vill bli jobbonär?* [Who wants to become a working retiree?] *MinPension.* https://blogg.minpension.se/

Whitehouse, E. (2007). *Life-expectancy risk and pensions: Who bears the burden?* (social, employment and migration working papers no. 60). OECD, Directorate for Employment, labour and social affairs. https://www.oecd.org/els/public-pensions/39469901.pdf

World Bank. (2003). *Lifelong learning in the global knowledge economy: Challenges for developing countries.* Directions in Development. https://openknowledge.worldbank.org/handle/10986/15141

World Bank. (2021, October). *Ending learning poverty and building skills: Investing in education from early childhood to lifelong learning* [Brochure]. https://thedocs.worldbank.org/en/doc/7b8e1ecfbeb0507559134a346bd64bc2-0200022022/related/WB-EducationBrochure-OCT-11-22-final-e-version-SP.pdf

World Bank. (2023). *Health nutrition and population statistics.* World Bank DataBank. https://databank.worldbank.org/source/health-nutrition-and-population-statistics#.

World Health Organization & European Observatory on Health Systems and Policies. (2021). *Promoting healthy ageing in the Western Pacific region: Implications for health expenditure trends and economic growth* [Policy brief]. https://eurohealthobservatory.who.int/publications/i/promoting-healthy-ageing-in-the-western-pacific-region-implications-for-health-expenditure-trends-and-economic-growth

Chapter 8
Lifelong Learning System

As early as Aristotle, learning was considered the best provision for successful aging. If that is the case, how can policies serve to extend lifelong learning for later life?

8.1 Major Changes Are Required for a True Lifelong Learning System

Successful societal requires adaptation to the type of change and dedication of time for the change process. Some changes are disruptive, shaking long established dominant ideas and restructuring frames of reference. They can cause the reversal of personal decisions, the launch of societal actions and the reshaping of relationships to others and society. Changes take time because the interrelationships between all elements need to be reoriented and harmonized. Citizens have to understand the new structures and plan how to use them to gain the expected benefits. Change rarely occurs in an isolated way, and people have to accept that multiple changes occur simultaneously but proceed at different speeds. Lifelong learning and technological change are examples. The order in which changes occur also matters, since change cannot always be legislated nor can a particular culture be imposed immediately.

S. Brink, *The Longevity Dividend*, International Perspectives on Aging 39,
https://doi.org/10.1007/978-3-031-35335-2_8

8.2 Do the Changes Required for Lifelong Learning Rank as a Paradigm Shift?

Learning will never be complete. Society must recognize learning as a lifelong necessity with multiple functions in modern life. Fundamental change alters the role of learning and how it is accessed during a long life. With time, lifelong learning permeates society beyond just the early adopters. When existing ideas are no longer compatible with lived experience, there may be some 'belief perseverance'. However, the shift in the thinking of the vast majority to adopt the new reality results in a paradigm shift (Kuhn, 1962).

A paradigm shift is a fundamental change which does not allow selecting favoured changes and ignoring others. To make lifelong learning a reality, systemic changes that are inter-related, multi-dimensional and simultaneous are required. Though the totality of change is unprecedented, there is no recommended path to making such a complex systemic change nor a strategy to make phased changes. But many existing program ideas and procedures can be used to further lifelong learning. Moreover, the speed of change can be managed, and leading societies will benefit from the 'first mover advantages' if they succeed earlier. Culture has to evolve around the changing learning system.

8.2.1 Policy Changes

The policy challenges are immense. The primary role of government would be to manage the asset of national human capital. If there is a minister of lifelong learning, he or she will have an enormous portfolio, since the learning of the entire population throughout life has to be directed for the progress of the country. New divisions of roles and responsibilities will evolve with the demands of the lifelong learning system. Government will have to manage through collaboration with multiple sectors, since many sectors of society and several professions will be involved in the lifelong learning system. Citizens will be responsible for their own learning but they will interact with many contacts in the system.

Lifelong learning will be both for public good and for private benefit. The democratization of learning will result in interaction with other public goods, such as health, standard of living and progress. The focus on the end user will be combined with the principle of subsidiarity, so that learners will access services from the organization closest to them. The exception will be remote learning but any mediator should be nearby or easily accessible. Public investments in learning have to be converted into equitably distributed relevant learning options for all ages, resulting in the growth and progress of the country. Governments will be held accountable by an educated population that is less likely to tolerate unfair inequities and more likely to protest the lack of social justice.

8.2.2 Organizational Changes

Learning will no longer be concentrated in initial education in the first quarter of life. This does not mean that established education provision will be abandoned. Rather, formal education between Kindergarten and Universities will be reformed to fit in a lifelong learning system. For example, education options will be made available for people of any age. Foundational skills (such as literacy, numeracy and learning-to-learn), once gained only in early life, will be learned continuously to support ongoing acquisition of knowledge. Higher education will no longer consist only of specialization and in-depth knowledge of a particular time but rather open to further development of knowledge, post graduation. Continuous learning of new ideas and evolving skills will be essential for coping with contemporary societal demands. Learning in every stage of life will have an important role, and each stage has to be integrated and consolidated with previous learning to form progressive options for the development of human capital. Organizational changes thus include interlinked options covering the life span rather than segments strictly specific to age and life stage. Learners should be able to access different levels of learning and utilize personalized pathways. Quality will be assessed by learning performance based on demonstrated competence and relevance to societal needs.

Learning options have to become wider and inter-linked, incorporating non-formal and informal learning. New forms of learning delivery, such as self-directed learning, open learning and digital learning, need to be incorporated integrally into the system. Learning could occur in multiple venues, not only in those dedicated solely to learning. Transdisciplinary combinations of disciplines, say, environmental law and biostatistics, will develop.

8.2.3 Financing a Lifelong Learning System

Financing lifelong learning in its entirety by a single sector is neither feasible nor practical. This follows from its long-term nature and because multiple stakeholders and actors are involved. Rather, an integrated lifelong learning system has to be financed jointly by multiple sources, such as private, public, professional or non-profit sectors, including individuals. Eligibility for incentives and subsidies will not be limited to particular age groups, or limited to specific places of learning. Financial instruments for lifelong saving and investments for education will be developed.

8.2.4 Attitudinal and Behavioural Changes

An illiterate person in the twenty-first century will be one who cannot learn, unlearn or relearn, as suggested by Toffler (1971). Learning will be impelled by continuous evaluation of the stock of personal knowledge in terms of its current relevance and the discarding of obsolete knowledge. Learning habits will be like those for health, which require continuous attention in daily life. There will be personal costs, such as loss of information and learning skill, if the process of knowledge accumulation is halted. In a lifelong learning culture, learning is an integral life function.

The process of learning will be reimagined. The differences between training and education will blur, because both require the acquisition of knowledge and skill. Learning can occur from a lecture, a demonstration video, a conversation with a mentor, a book, a short course, a work placement or an education program.

While learning is a right of citizenship, with a return on personal investment and a share of social benefits, it also implies individual responsibilities. Learning is a shared responsibility with other citizens and actors in education, such as the state, institutions, educators and the media. Nonetheless, learning is voluntary. Returns will be dependent on learning agency.

8.3 National Experiments with Learning Account Programs Have Transferable Elements for Lifelong Learning

Various policy designs for learning account programs can pave the way for lifelong learning. Several countries and other jurisdictions have run pilots or experimental programs with learning accounts. They include United Kingdom (Individual Learning Accounts), Canada (learn$ave., Lifelong Learning Plan), France (*Compte personnel de formation*), Singapore (SkillsFuture Credit), states of Washington and Michigan (Individual Learning Accounts), Upper Austria (*Bildungskonto*), Tuscany (*Carta ILA*), and Scotland (Individual Learning Accounts and Individual Training Accounts) (OECD, 2019; Perez & Vourc'h, 2020). Although none of these programs extended to old age, some of their characteristics may have value for the organization and management of lifelong learning.

The programs had characteristics involving some of the following elements. First, statutory right to learning while working or in retirement through a personal learning plan or account. Second, individual responsibility and initiative for managing lifelong learning. Third, individual choice of content to meet personal needs, preferred time and length of learning and the appropriate provider. Fourth, access to learning with portability across disciplines, jobs and location. Fifth, involvement of multiple actors, such as individuals, governments, savings institutions, employers, trade unions, community organizations, professionals, and others. Sixth, incentives such as advantageous savings instruments, tax benefits, targeted subsidies (for low-income learners, for example) and discount vouchers for priority skills in demand in the labour market. Seventh, minimization of disincentives, such as replacing lost earnings during learning. Eighth, preferential access to longer knowledge and skills programs (not superficial or recreation/leisure programs) resulting in diploma, certification or license or skill guarantee. Ninth, professional assessment and consultation on ideal learning options incorporated into learning plans.

8.4 Lifelong Learning Requires New Thinking About Building Human Capital

Successfully implementing a lifelong learning system within a relatively short time is a challenge. National governments have experience managing public goods for their citizens. Thus far education has been such a policy field. However, past experience, institutions and structures are less helpful when implementing lifelong learning. This is because knowledge itself has undergone a major change.

8.4.1 Knowledge as Public Goods

Knowledge that is constantly evolving and is available worldwide can be considered a 'global public good'. It potentially offers benefits to all people of many generations in all countries. To be successful, learning has to be of a global standard and be up to date. Lifelong learning is the means to achieving this. Global public goods have three features. They are non-rivalrous, where consumption by anybody does not reduce the quantity available to others. They are non-excludable, meaning that it is impossible to prevent or prohibit anyone from consuming it. They are potentially globally available, despite limiting conditions (Stiglitz, 1999). The public goods nature of lifelong learning underpins a global interest in developing policies for lifelong learning at every level in order to reinforce the knowledge infrastructure.

There are challenges associated with global public knowledge, however. Knowledge of various quality is produced and consumed at various rates all around the world. Though globally available, it is unevenly distributed and learned. While globally valuable, it may need to be adapted to the place and time where it will be used. To gain maximum value, knowledge has to be accessed and learned continually by as many people as possible. These global flows of knowledge through lifelong learning are critical for world progress and a key means to reduce inequities between and within countries. The internet has been an important vehicle for the free spread of knowledge around the world. Nonetheless, governments have a role in ensuring that their citizens are capable of learning and accessing global current knowledge throughout life.

The benefits of societal learning are based not only on national human capital but also on new knowledge creation. Both of these have international ramifications as countries collaborate and compete for economic advantage. National economies can be driven by knowledge, by a labour force with competencies based on knowledge and by high value production where knowledge is embedded.

8.4.2 Lifelong Learning Is a Strategy for a Learning Society

Lifelong learning is a broad, generic term in use for a decade or two. Since it is popularly used loosely also to describe related concepts, such as adult learning or training, it is difficult to convey its critical role to the general public. Moreover, its role is often linked to other concepts, such as the learning economy and the learning society. Simply put, members of a learning society build human capital through lifelong learning in order to develop knowledge workers and consumers that work to grow a learning economy driven by knowledge.

Lifelong learning involves a continuously evolving learning system, which serves all life stages in each generation. The lifelong learning system is responsible for a lifetime of learning. Learning at some stages is well advanced but poorly developed in others, often in later life. These weaker links reduce the benefit flow from knowledge throughout life. Well curated and accumulated learning can achieve the greater good through improved capacity to contribute to a learning society – something larger and more enduring than benefits to one individual during a lifetime.

Learning as a part of life is a new idea. People often indulge in incidental and informal learning without seeking to maximize its value for their human capital. Conscious and intentional learning is a life skill that needs to be fostered.

8.4.3 Lifelong Learning as a Policy Domain

Establishing lifelong learning will challenge traditional policy making because it is a universal entitlement or right based in law but it is also a public benefit that requires structure and organization. Protection of the right may be simpler than practical demands for national delivery of learning over a life a time. Many policy principles such as accountability, equal treatment and equitable results may require modified application.

Having to manage an equitable distribution of knowledge in a context of abundance, rather than scarcity, seems paradoxical. It is also new to contend with misinformation, fake news and weaponizing of knowledge. Learning is distributed in new and multiple ways, including through digital technologies and unprecedented connectivity. Knowledge changes quickly, which requires strategies for sorting by relevance for consolidation, integration and transmission.

Ensuring public accountability for policy outcomes can be problematic, since outcomes can vary with age, context and competencies learned. Developing, distributing, monitoring and evaluating policies for lifelong learning may require new policy solutions. Lifelong learning policies may need to be different from current policy approaches in new previously untried ways.

Each stage of life has its specific needs and demand for the content and types of learning, which are modified by the context. Learning as a preschooler differs from that of an adult. With age, one's learning needs diversify, and customization covers different types of learning, such as formal, informal, digital learning, and peer learning. It can even include unlearning to discard obsolete learning. Learning objectives can be based on content. However, learning processes cannot be standardized for all ages, nor can they be easily specified by the place, time or method to acquire knowledge and skills.

Equity can be a key part of public policy. However, pursuing equity makes it more difficult to customize learning. Customization must allow for variable speeds of learning and choice of components through life. Individual learners may acquire the same learning by different processes over varying periods of time at different stages of life.

The rapid changes in knowledge contents and how it is delivered will make accreditation challenging. Microlearning with certification or badges for shorter sub-components that can be combined in different ways may be part of the solution.

Lifelong learning links past learning with learning for the future. The cumulated aggregate human capital has greater value than exceptional performance in one stage of life. Therefore, lifelong learning may need to be evaluated intermittently during its progress. Approbation could be conferred at intermediate steps, based on continuous monitoring, instead of once at termination, such as graduation from university.

8.4.4 Reliable Evidence Based on Accurate Measurements Is Required to Assess the Success of the Design and Implementation of Lifelong Learning Policies

The design and implementation of policies is always arduous but more so during periods of transition. Policy design should be based on evidence, but it is not always available or stable during periods of change. Likewise, though evidence of the value of lifelong learning is solid, parameters for its implementation are neither stable nor traditional. The design and implementation of policies thus face a variety of challenges.

The participation of an individual in lifelong learning is not always specific in relation to time, domain or activity, and assessments are difficult to administer and to measure. Outcomes must measure learning performance unrelated to the method or time used to learn. Experience with Prior Learning Assessment and Recognition (PLAR) might provide useful procedures.

Measuring the impact of policies is difficult if expected outcomes are not clearly defined. For example, in today's knowledge economy, there is no clear separation between knowledge producers and knowledge consumers. The line between these activities is increasingly indistinct and each individual is expected to engage both in productive use of human capital and in co-creation of knowledge with others.

Policies are usually designed to treat individuals the same. However, the needs for learning are diverse as each individual develops from childhood to old age. This diversity in needs for learning is valuable for enriching societal human capital. To complement the traditional standardized measurements, the development of better ways to measure diversity and personalization would stimulate innovation in learning.

Chosen measurements of policy performance are usually stable over the duration of the policy. However, the flows of information are not static over time, so measurements need to be relative and adaptable. They may need to be adjusted in relation to the speed of knowledge creation and the exposure of individuals to knowledge during the years of policy implementation. Individuals receive a flood of information, and their capacity to absorb information is subject to individual variation. The metrics used for learning curricula therefore have to be continually adjusted. An hour of learning is not necessarily comparable across learners.

The effectiveness of policies can be evaluated periodically during implementation and checked against the context of demands of the time for midcourse corrections. Poor or slow implementation of policies can make them fall short of delivering the intended result. Evaluation of policies to gauge their result therefore sometimes takes place only after a decade of implementation.

8.4.5 Policies for Lifelong Learning Have to Rely on Partnership with Individuals

No citizen is in theory excluded from lifelong learning. The attitude of the general public therefore influences the design and enactment of policies. Policies can be designed to be universal but may be deemed successful only if a majority of citizens participate fairly steadily without legal coercion. Lack of, or only intermittent, participation throughout life can negatively affect the achievement of maximum individual and national benefits. Achieving full participation all the time by everyone in lifelong learning may be difficult since it is a relatively new policy endeavour. This is especially so if people in some life stages, such as later life, see little reason to engage.

8.5 The Public Policy Challenge

The need for lifelong learning has been acknowledged by governments since the 1990s. It would be disastrous for a country to offer no possibilities for lifelong learning. Progress has been slow and uneven as policies have been made, abandoned and redesigned while searching for the best solutions. Since lifelong learning is seen as everyone's shared responsibility, it is difficult to assign responsibility and accountability.

Public policy making has been described as the art of the possible. Public policy is whatever governments choose to do or not do in order to achieve an intended purpose. Some policies are required by international law, such as those related to rights. A policy goal is usually to achieve a widely accepted outcome, sometimes agreed upon after wide public consultation and discussion. A policy guides decisions along an intentional course of action, adopted by governments, institutions, businesses, groups of individuals or individual citizens or all of them together, to achieve that outcome. There can be competing or even controversial views of how knowledge is to be used for social progress. Such differences affect how knowledge is created, used and disseminated in society. With a widely agreed goal, criteria can be developed to help judge the merits of competing courses of action. Criteria can relate to, for example, ensuring the best outcome for the most people with the least negative impact or risk of unintended consequences. A policy that effectively and efficiently provides the greatest good, for the longest time, for the most people at the least cost would be judged as successful.

What are the potential government policy levers for implementing lifelong learning? Policies can lead, govern, forbid, regulate, encourage and incentivize actions by people to engage in lifelong learning. Table 8.1 identifies some useful attributes of the potential government roles for lifelong learning.

8.6 Infrastructures for Learning in the Later Years

Often motivated by intellectual curiosity, people in their later years rely on lifelong learning opportunities to learn new things for pleasure, to understand their life-world context, to improve the quality of their own life and to participate in society. It might even be hypothesized that the widest range of learning content would be required for the later years because the needs and experience of those learners are very diverse. The demand for formal, non-formal, informal and digital learning is to some extent met by specialized arrangements, such as lifelong learning institutes and Universities of the Third Age in several countries (Phillipson & Ogg, 2010). Social institutions, such as churches, clubs, community centres and folk schools have widened their array of programming by adding learning opportunities for older learners (Findsen, 2006). Learning opportunities are also provided for residents in care homes and nursing homes. Having more older people than children in a country

Table 8.1 Potential government policy roles for lifelong learning

Policy lever	Example potential policy actions for lifelong learning
Leadership	Make national pronouncements about vision and goals; facilitate the creation of missing or weak components of lifelong learning such as late life learning; stable efforts for long-term policy.
Co-ordinator	Integrate multi-sectoral lifelong learning provision by other actors such as municipalities, learning institutions, unions, employers, private companies, etc.
Interlocutor	Public consultations and consensus building; manage relationships with international organizations, other countries, competitors; mediate issues; create networks.
Intergovernmental linkage	Alignment between multilateral government efforts for lifelong learning; facilitate exchanges; sharing of resources.
Inform and educate	Exhort universal participation while explaining life altering benefits; publicize opportunities; public information campaigns; highlight success stories.
Evidence generation	Create evidence to support decision making by all actors; collect data, conduct and finance research; synthesize research from relevant sources; knowledge mobilization; regular dissemination of research results; knowledge consolidation over time.
Assuror	Assure the provision of choice and opportunities for all stages of life.
Quality assurance	Standards of provision, credentials, proficiency recognition; consumer protection: ensure a reasonable return on investment (fees, time, effort).
Funder	Cost sharing with other levels of government; incentives to create a diversity of providers; grants and subsidies to learners.
Operations	Operate public institutions; conduct learning programs of all types to demonstrate a new component or to fill gaps in the system.

Author's elaboration from Brink (2008)

requires managing the structures and resources appropriately for meeting learning needs throughout life.

8.7 Suggested Indicators for an Ideal Lifelong Learning System

Education exists as an already composite sector that involves a great number of people and institutions. It also addresses learning in fairly well delineated parts – early childhood education, compulsory schooling, higher education, vocational education, work related training, etc. Lifelong long learning adds complexity but it integrates the different aspects of learning and creates a system.

Not all parts of the existing system will be affected in the same way by a shift to lifelong learning. The shift is nonetheless a major transformative change, which requires acceptance of non-traditional learning pathways, new ways of learning and learning throughout life. Both equity and excellence parameters need to be met for the full benefits of lifelong learning to be achieved. Countries need to be able to convert education and learning into social progress for all, not just for an elite or a young segment of the population.

Countries vary in the way they develop their lifelong learning systems, but there are also commonalities. A country may see a need to examine its existing or evolving lifelong learning system, identify gaps and set objectives for improvement. In so shaping its own system, a country may find it useful to evaluate its progress by using a checklist (as follows) based on the characteristics of an ideal lifelong learning system.

8.7.1 Lifelong Learning Systemic Factors

While system components such as preschool education have special characteristics, the lifelong learning system deals with the entire population with its diverse demands and at all ages.

- *A functional lifelong learning system is comprehensive and reticulated*

The education system has been compartmentalized, linear and cumulative so far. The lifelong learning system functions best if it is more web-like, offering multiple pathways in different directions. Individuals will have the chance to build their own personal pathways of learning that start at any point, depending on their personal challenges and opportunities as they proceed through life. Opportunities should be tailored to meeting the changing needs and demands at all stages of life whenever they occur.

- *Interrelationship of components*

Lifelong learning needs a structure that is complicated because its many components are managed by different sectors of society. Some examples are public, private, non-profit entities, educational institutions, social organizations, labour unions, and various communities. They need to work in sync to achieve the desired results. Poor linkages and weak collaboration can be detrimental to the whole system. Lifelong learning requires a systemic approach for the success of each component as well as the whole.

- *Coordination mechanism*

A national coordination mechanism is essential to ensure that the components work as a system and serve multiple stakeholders effectively. The coordination mechanism can be designed to suit each country but it should be composed of government ministries, employers, workers, professionals, learners and other stakeholders. It could be an independent advisory body to parliament or to a cabinet committee for lifelong learning. SITRA in Finland is an example of an independent multi-stakeholder advisory body.

- *Lifelong learning includes multiple objectives*

Learning can be driven by different objectives, singly or in combination, during the lifetime. All of the objectives are recognized as valid, whether it is self-development, increased human capital, mastery of life skills or understanding societal challenges.

- *Allocation of funding*

All components of lifelong learning should be fairly and adequately funded, so as to ensure equitable access to all throughout their lives. Funding should be adequate for the potential size of the demand and its projected growth.

8.7.2 Lifelong Learning Processes

- *Permeable and inter-related components*

Less segmentation and more links allow the components to create a larger number and combinations of future options. The components should have porous boundaries that allow them to accept new non-traditional learners. Each component should offer learning through different modes and be adaptable for different age and ability groups. The components should nonetheless be efficient within their boundaries to achieve quality learning.

- *Personalized pathways*

It should be possible for individuals to remedy learning gaps and delays and missed or forgotten learning. This means that pathways cannot be linear and unidirectional. It should be acceptable for someone to go back to learning parts that are missing in their human capital, whatever the reason for the shortfall. It should be possible to enter the system at multiple points and to design a personalized package of learning options with a choice of start and end points. Personalized pathways may be multi-directional and divergent. A choice of a learning option should not limit future choices and previous events should not constrain future pathways. Open Universities offer learners course options to create their own program.

- *Access to learning opportunities*

Access assures equal and equitable opportunities for learning at every stage of life. Ensuring access to learning opportunities is difficult because, over time, learners are at different points in their own learning journeys, with different assets and difficulties in their lives. Facilitating access is not as simple as providing additional spaces, financial assistance or a multiplicity of providers. Making access realistic includes accommodating a diversity of learning needs, such as the provision of pre-requisites, remedial learning and varying times for completion.

- *Multiple ways of learning, resulting in comparable competencies*

Learning may be formal, non-formal or informal. It can be digital, teacher led, learning from peers or self-directed. Learning can be in a class or a group setting.

Learning can result through work or through internships and apprenticeships. Appropriate and blended pedagogies should be used for best learning results. The focus is not on where or how learning occurs but rather on what competencies are gained. Frequently revised national standards of competencies should be accepted by all employers and education providers.

- *Guidance and counselling*

Guidance and counselling services, national if possible, could help people to navigate the complex learning system, suggest appropriate options, inform about local availability and help with the development of learning portfolios (see below). The options should include formal, non-formal, informal and digital learning. This could also be a location for collection and storage of data on participation in the identified learning options.

- *Places for learning*

While dedicated institutions for learning are necessary, learning should also be encouraged in all places where knowledge is developed, taught, learned, shared or used. These could be non-traditional spaces (a prison, for instance) or multiuse spaces such as a libraries, hospitals, community centres or theatres. The key is to offer places to which learners have easy access, by foot or public transportation.

- *Recognition of qualifications and competencies*

Qualifications should be standardized in meaningful ways, both to enable the learner to value them and to signal the learner's competencies to others. Aggregated information on standardized competencies serves numerous purposes, such as estimating demand for further education to meet developments in the labour market or for societal standing. Learning outcomes, regardless of the way they were acquired, should be described in ways that are portable. This means they have to be up-to-date so they continue to function as job markets change or individuals face challenges in life. Credentials attesting to learning outcomes can take a variety of forms such as diplomas, certificates and badges, registered by the issuing body. For a particular competency, the standard used by a specific credential should be known and be comparable to other qualifications. Such qualifications should be transparent for both the learner and others.

The flexibility and transferability of knowledge and skills as well as transdisciplinary knowledge should be recognized. It should be possible to transfer previously learned competencies when retraining or upskilling or switching disciplines.

- *Quality assurance through assessments*

Multiple types of assessments should be used to measure progress of individual learners and to monitor equity and efficiency of results in and among groups. Returns to learning vary over time, and they need to be continually monitored. Assessments should be regularly updated to stay current with the demands of real life. Assessment metrics have a role not only in serving labour market needs but also for individuals' participation in society, self-care and autonomy, culture and citizenship.

- *Individual portfolios of learning*

Portfolios of learning are sometimes called human capital accounts. A personal portfolio keeps track of acquisition, obsolescence and progressive width and extent of growth in knowledge and competencies for personal use. It communicates one's learning stock to others, such as employers. Such portfolios or accounts can help individuals to make decisions, based on returns to learning, about further investments based on content, time and effort. Transparency in accounting facilitates a person's progression over time and comparison with the qualifications of others. It can also identify a person's unique combinations of skills of value. Each annual investment in learning is recognized.

8.7.3 Lifelong Learning Actors

- *Individual learners*

The centrality of the learner is significant. Individuals have responsibility for their own learning, and they need to invest in learning through the life span in order to maximize their potential. They are expected to display agency, acting independently to exercise their own choice to avert the risk of lowering their potential or their quality of life. Learning is no longer attached more to some stages of life than to others. Rather, learning is an integral part of life, similar to healthy habits and fiscal prudence. Individuals must prepare themselves with foundational skills, such as literacy and numeracy, and 'learning-to-learn' skills. Although learning is voluntary and self-directed, responsible decisions about lifelong learning are necessary to manage the demands of life. Lifelong learning is, however, a shared responsibility, so a failure to learn cannot be attributed solely to the individual. When a society does not encourage lifelong learning for all, it accepts a lower return from national human capital.

- *Stakeholders*

When everyone is a lifelong learner, everyone is not only a stakeholder in their own learning but also a stakeholder in the learning of others. Peer learning and intergenerational learning involve learning by all participants. Benefits accrue to all individuals living in a society with high human capital. Many other citizen roles have a stake in human capital. For example, parents have a stake in the learning of their children, employers of their workers and unions of their members.

- *Education professionals*

Distributing knowledge and managing equitable returns to learning are among the main tasks of society. While learning is a complex social activity, it can be facilitated by professionals trained in the learning sciences specific to special needs and specific demands of life. Proper training handles both the subjects of specialization and the pedagogy of successful learning. For instance, early childhood educators specialize in the learning of young children and pedagogies related to play. Planning the supply to meet current and future demand or shortages in various areas of education is essential. This can include, for example, geragogy for people in their later years.

- *Providers of lifelong learning*

Whether public, private or non-profit, providers of lifelong learning are major actors. They are responsible for the relevance of learning programs and learning outcomes as knowledge becomes the medium of exchange in learning economies and societies. As major players in the system providers have a stake in its success. The opportunities for learning have to be diverse and attractive to learners. Lifelong learning opens opportunities for diversification and increases in the provision of learning through competition for learners.

- *Knowledge producers*

Researchers, designers and inventors are vested in the knowledge economy and society. The learning system is a major vehicle for the dissemination of new knowledge.

- *Governments*

Governments are major stakeholders as they play multiple roles in the learning system (Table 8.1). They also benefit from lifelong learning. Educated countries have better governance, rule of law and less corruption because citizens understand issues, engage in the political process and hold their governments accountable (Lurie, 2014).

8.7.4 Learning Resources

- *Learning resources and supports*

Knowledge is increasing at a tremendously fast pace, so learning resources must be continuously updated. Annual updating of digital learning materials may be an option. It is also critical to modernize the ways to produce learning resources and to use them for lifelong learning. Additional resources, such as tutoring, may be necessary for individuals with difficulties learning.

- *Technology for knowledge dissemination*

Technology is a ubiquitous and growing resource in present day life. People receive information at home and elsewhere through a large and changing variety of digital streams on many kinds of electronic devices, in addition to traditional media such as radio, television and print. The number of internet users in the world could be 5.3 billion in 2023, which is almost two-thirds of the world population (International Telecommunication Union, 2023). Digital devices in conjunction with suitable content generation can be not only a tool for dissemination of created knowledge products, such as blogs, but also a medium for formal and informal learning activity. New technologies should be considered for use in pedagogy. For example, artificial intelligence and virtual reality are being tested for tailor made learning for a digital community of learners and for personal tutoring.

- *Open Educational Resources (OER)*

OER have enlarged the learning opportunities by providing alternate and enhanced resources that are freely available. These are teaching, learning and research materials in any medium – digital or otherwise. They reside in the public domain or have been released under an open license that permits no-cost access, use, adaptation and redistribution by others with no or only limited restrictions.

The right to use OER freely is valuable for late-life learners. This right enables them to integrate learned information by reusing and revising it to conform and enlarge their prior learning and experience. They enrich the learning by remixing it with other related pieces of information and retaining it in their memory. They may create new information and share it with others, in addition to sharing the original information in the OER (Wiley & Hilton, 2018).

8.7.5 Financing Lifelong Learning

- *Investing in lifelong learning*

While learning is a cost of modern life it is also an investment. The learning economy depends on investment to ensure knowledge is produced, consumed and applied. Such investment is part of the cost of living and of doing business. For example, employers may provide time away from work for the purpose of learning. The learning society adopts it as a legitimate cost of living expenditure. Public policy can include investment in institutions, personnel, data and research. Policy incentives and disincentives can steer lifelong learning activities. Disadvantaged learners can be subsidized by financial assistance or low interest loans, and meritorious learners can be offered scholarships and grants.

- *Co-financing*

Lifelong learning involves multiple sectors in order to support learning by the entire population. Co-financing by public, private and non-public sectors as well as by individuals makes this possible. A strategy of collaborative financing is valuable as it manifests the joint commitment of stakeholders. For instance, banks can support public tax incentives in savings programs, while individuals can engage in saving for learning.

8.7.6 Policy Mix

- *Policies for lifelong learning*

A lifelong learning policy is an overarching policy under which inter-linked component policies can be accommodated. Educational reform is required to transform from life-stage based learning to lifelong learning while retaining the best of the existing system.

Lessons can be learned from national health policy and its infrastructure. For instance, a learning card can be issued to citizens for life, where every interaction with the learning system is recorded showing the learning trajectory. Regular interactions with the system would be expected (similar to health checkups and annual vaccinations). When the system is entered, a person's need is evaluated regardless of age and he or she is directed to the right discipline and organization to meet that need. This is similar to when one enters a general hospital. If multiple disciplines are needed, then multiple specialists can work together in the most appropriate way to meet the need. Perhaps a list of choices can be provided. A person leaves the learning system when the need is met, with suggestions of further actions at home.

Introducing and managing such a large-scale transition is an important responsibility, because there can be grave consequences if groups of people are left out and if learning by future generations is affected. Policies that are incompatible with lifelong learning must be dropped, revised or reformulated, and new policies must be developed according to need. Long term policies should ensure that people's learning careers are not subject to interruptions or rapid changes, which could even disrupt their lives.

- *Policy evaluation, policy coordination and evidence-based policy reform*

During the transformation to lifelong learning, it is important to examine each individual policy for its specific contribution to the whole. It is at the same time essential to review the entire comprehensive policy mix to check that it is cohesive and provides the expected result on a population-wide scale. Policy evaluation has to be detailed enough to discover any failing. For example, the policy may be ineffective, poorly designed or poorly implemented or the components may be badly coordinated.

The evaluation has to look at policy success both horizontally, at a given point in time, and longitudinally over time. This makes it possible to identify any weak link in the course of lifelong learning. The evidence from the evaluation should articulate whether the policy response is sufficient to sustain people's motivation to keep learning throughout their lives. Possibilities for policy reform need to be built-in to make policy combinations flexible enough to adapt to changes in demand in the future. Evaluation of outcomes should be the reason for policy change, and policy analysis based on data should underpin policy reform.

- *Data needs for planning and policy development*

National human capital stocks and flows need to be measured, and findings need to be shared. For forward planning, a government needs to know the evolving demand for knowledge and skills and also the type and extent of any surpluses and shortages. Building expertise and experience takes time, which means that planning needs to be continuous. Having data only from formal learning institutions is insufficient. Data on where people learn, what they learn, and how well they have learned is essential. Policies need to ensure that people are guided to learning that will be of value to them. Soft persuasion, such as encouragement, incentives, public promotion and recognition, can encourage learning.

- *Research in education and human capital*

Fine-grained research should examine the learning process of individuals at every age, including the later years, and the progression of learning through life. Segmenting the population helps to understand the different variables affecting their learning. Understanding the effects of intersectionality make it possible to ensure that equity is achieved throughout life. Over-the-horizon issues should be on the research agenda, since they will alter demand. Examples include the emerging areas of knowledge, the impact of future technology and the relationship between knowledge and progress.

8.7.7 A Culture that Favours Lifelong Learning

- *Embedding learning in culture*

Culture has been called the way of life for an entire society. A culture of lifelong learning can thus be described as a widely accepted life-steering collection of values and attitudes, which generates lifelong learning activities in the population (OECD, 2010). When learning and sharing of knowledge are embedded in culture, they are normal everyday human activities. Children are socialized to include learning as a life activity. The culture promotes a systemic view of learning and creates a shared responsibility for its success.

8.8 Mutual Responsibilities of All Actors

All actors involved in lifelong learning have many shared and mutual responsibilities. They include agency, good practices of knowledge management, integration of the system, co-ordination and collaboration, policy and costs of lifelong learning. The responsibilities of these actors are linked to their primary role within the lifelong learning system, with the understanding that poor performance of one affects the system as a whole. Since responsibilities are shared, each actor is accountable for the success or failure of not only the outcomes of others but also that of the system. This means each actor has to cooperate and collaborate with other components and other actors. Table 8.2 describes the kinds of mutual responsibilities of the different actors.

8.9 A Learning Society or a Learning Divide?

The rationale for the introduction of learning societies was that change is constant in modern times, and adapting to this changing condition requires constant learning (Schön, 1973). Lifelong learning and learning societies are mutually dependent. Lifelong learning is necessary to replenish and improve knowledge and skills to create desirable futures for individuals and societies.

A learning society is a collective in which all members contribute to the learning, sharing and construction of knowledge continually throughout their lives. Consequently, all members gain the resulting benefits of prosperity, quality of life and wellbeing. However, all members of society may not all benefit equally from learning or enjoy the benefits of the learning society. The learning divide is the gap between learners and non-learners, whatever the reason for their non-participation.

Older people in later life are at high risk of being non-learners and therefore being excluded and left behind. There are indications that learning participation falls steeply in the later years (Fig. 8.1). In other cases, learning is limited or inadequate. This may be because learning on topics of importance in later life, such as pensions, will and testament preparation or falls prevention, are not available.

People are living longer but that is no reason for them to cease learning. Lifelong learning implies that learning is accumulated over the lifetime, which improves, corrects and updates knowledge and experience. The benefits gained by the individual and society will depend on what and how much the individual learns by continuous learning, including in the later years.

Continual learning gains enable a person to cope with the unpredictable challenges of life and to take advantage of opportunities to control their personal destiny. Continued learning increases the person's real capacity to contribute to current society and to transmit experience and ideas to prepare the younger generation for their future lives. A society of learners is a productive society.

If no learning takes place, the losses are real. To not continue to learn is to decline in personal wellbeing. There are losses of literacy and learning skills from disuse. Since this results in poor or no learning, a person's human capital could include obsolete skills in the repertoire and knowledge that is no longer useful. Further, the lack of learning of current knowledge and skills (digital skills, for example) is a lost opportunity. Life expectancy can be reduced both by a lack of knowledge gains and by mounting knowledge losses. Society also loses in a competitive world, since its human capital is less than it could be.

Table 8.2 Mutual responsibilities of the actors in the lifelong learning system

Areas of responsibility	Governments	Institutions, providers	Professionals	Individuals and families
Agency	Leadership in the provision of lifelong learning for national progress and economic growth.	Managing the transformation to lifelong learning, while ensuring personalization for diversity of learners.	Focus on appropriate pedagogies for developing competencies in a lifelong learning framework.	Self-direction, independence and commitment to lifelong learning for personal and social benefit.
Good practices of knowledge management	Production of national data, aggregator of research information, repository of evolving knowledge and national dissemination of knowledge as needed.	Testing of hypotheses or published information, creation of knowledge through research, synthesis of research, packaging of information for education according to need, dissemination to wider public.	Knowledge managers and brokers, packaging knowledge for learning, linking it to application and daily experience.	Searching for knowledge, evaluating its accuracy and value, interpretation and integration, understanding its potential use in relevant situations, sharing information where appropriate with other learners or within the family.
Integration of a system based on lifelong learning	Ensuring a lifelong learning system, integrating its components.	Specific role within the system and integration with other parts.	Integration of knowledge for transdisciplinary competences for flexibility and portability.	Integration of learning and continual checks with reality for relevance.
Coordination and collaboration	Coordination of components and multilateral collaboration between levels of government and institutions.	Coordination and collaboration within and between institutions to ensure quality and equity of provision.	Collaboration between knowledge producers and educators nationally and internationally to ensure relevance and efficacy.	Coordination of life responsibilities and management of effort and time for lifelong learning of individuals and family members.

(continued)

Table 8.2 (continued)

Areas of responsibility	Governments	Institutions, providers	Professionals	Individuals and families
Policy	Policies based on evidence to ensure efficiency, excellence and equity; national multisectoral overview for linkages between taxes, labour market, social wellbeing and human capital; consumer protection, quality assurance and guarantee of the qualification granted.	Effective use of national and local data to create institutional policies to ensure quality provision of learning, use of institutional data to monitor quality and performance.	Professional policies for quality of practice, continual professional updating and training.	Personal policies for commitment to lifelong learning, socialization and preparation of children for lifelong learning.
Costs of lifelong learning	Infrastructure support; tax subsidies to donors to education and non-profit organizations providing education; provision of incentives and disincentives, such as tax benefits and tax credits, vouchers, subsidies; loans and grants for those in financial need.	Prudent fiscal management of provision and best use of government support; cost sharing where possible through fee reduction, scholarships for learners, supports to professionals for in-service training, such as leave, financial support or special instruction and group learning.	Efficient use of resources to ensure the best learning outcomes and results for future learning; use of incentives for continuous learning and training; active participation in professional settings to advance professional knowledge and pedagogical know how to get best results for cost.	Use of tax-sheltered saving for education, incentives and disincentives such as tax credits, vouchers, subsidies, loans and grants; equitable usage of resources for members of the family to ensure lifelong learning.

Author's elaboration, 2023

8.10 Later Lives Are Enhanced by Lifelong Learning

Lifelong learning must be lifelong in reality. Learning is an essential part of life because knowledge is vital for quality of life and for participation in and contribution to society throughout life. Lifelong learning enables individuals to become and be the persons they aspire to be and to do the things they value, while contributing to society and to future generations. The democratization of knowledge through lifelong learning ensures that everyone has the knowledge required to make the

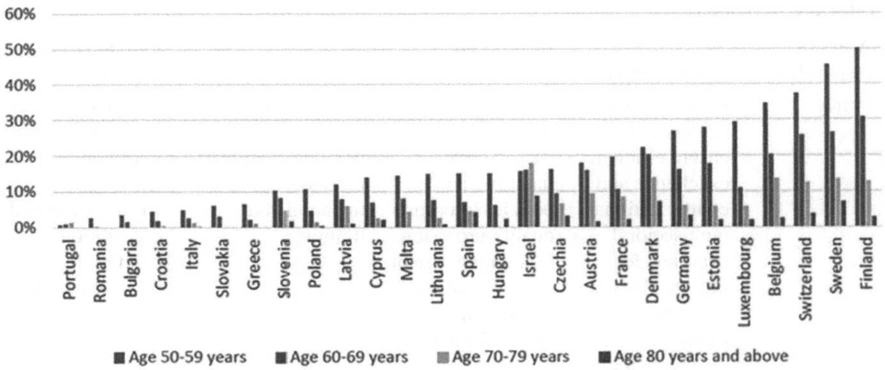

Fig. 8.1 Participation in learning declines with age, selected countries, 2021. (Reproduced from Lifelong learning in ageing societies: Lessons from Europe by Ogg (2021, Figure 3, Percentage of older people who attended an educational or training course in the preceding year) (analysis based on data from the Survey of Health, Ageing and Retirement in Europe (n.d.)) with permission from UNESCO Institute for Lifelong Learning)

most of the opportunities offered by their lives. This process should not stop in later life, especially with a growing lifespan.

People in later life comprise a sizeable and growing segment of the population, and their contributions are important for the progress of society. In turn, society should invest in people throughout their lives by enabling lifelong learning. Wellbeing over the lifetime is a societal goal, and lifelong learning ensures that the specific needs of each stage of life can be met in a way that makes a long life worth living. There is evidence that living in a democratic country can add up to 11 years to one's life expectancy (Patterson & Veenstra, 2016). This suggests the presence of a fair social compact for learning by people of all ages, including those in their later years.

References

Brink, S. (2008, June 24–27). *Lifelong learning – The role of public policy* [Unpublished paper]. Leveraging Learning for Regional Development: An International Forum. Lakehead University, Thunder Bay, Ontario.

Findsen, B. (2006). Social institutions as sites of learning for older adults: Differential opportunities. *Journal of Transformative Education, 4*(1), 65–81. https://doi.org/10.1177/1541344605282429

International Telecommunication Union. (2023, January 26). *Statistics*. https://www.itu.int/en/ITU-D/Statistics/Pages/stat/default.aspx

Kuhn, T. S. (1962). *The structure of scientific revolutions*. University of Chicago Press.

Lurie, S. (2014, March 6). Highly educated countries have better governments. *The Atlantic*. https://www.theatlantic.com/education/archive/2014/03/highly-educated-countries-have-better-governments/284273/

OECD. (2010). *PISA 2009 results: What students know and can do – Student performance in reading, mathematics and science (Volume I)*. https://doi.org/10.1787/9789264091450-en

OECD. (2019). *Individual learning accounts: Panacea or pandora's box?* https://doi.org/10.1787/203b21a8-en

Ogg, J. (2021). *Lifelong learning in ageing societies: Lessons from Europe*. Commissioned for *Embracing a culture of lifelong learning*, the UNESCO Institute for Lifelong Learning's contribution to UNESCO's Futures of Education initiative. https://unesdoc.unesco.org/ark:/48223/pf0000377820

Patterson, A. C., & Veenstra, G. (2016). Politics and population health: Testing the impact of electoral democracy. *Health & Place, 40*(July), 66–75. https://doi.org/10.1016/j.healthplace.2016.04.011

Perez, C., & Vourc'h, A. (2020). *Individualising training access schemes: France – The Compte Personnel de Formation (Personal Training Account – CPF)* (OECD social, employment and migration working papers no. 245). OECD. https://doi.org/10.1787/301041f1-en

Phillipson, C., & Ogg, J. (2010). *Active ageing and universities: Engaging older learners* (Research report). Universities UK. https://dera.ioe.ac.uk/26269/1/ActiveAgeing.pdf

Schön, D. A. (1973). *Beyond the stable state: Public and private learning in a changing society*. Penguin.

Stiglitz, J. E. (1999). Knowledge as global public good. In I. Kaul, I. Grunberg, & M. A. Stern (Eds.), *Global public goods: International cooperation in the 21st century* (pp. 308–325). Oxford University Press.

Survey of Health, Ageing and Retirement in Europe. (n.d.). *SHARE-ERIC* [Data portal]. https://share-eric.eu/

Toffler, A. (1971). *Future shock*. Bantam Books.

Wiley, D., & Hilton, J. (2018). Defining OER-enabled pedagogy. *International Review of Research in Open and Distributed Learning, 19*(4), 133–147. https://doi.org/10.19173/irrodl.v19i4.3601

Chapter 9
Lifelong Learning and the Social Compact

'Society is indeed a contract,' wrote Edmund Burke, the British Parliamentarian, more than two centuries ago. 'It becomes a partnership not only between those who are living, but between those who are living, those who are dead, and those who are to be born.' (Burke, 1790). Compared to the sharing of other societal assets, this description most aptly describes the social compact or contract covering shared ownership and free transfers of knowledge for the advancement of society.

9.1 The Social Compact

The Oxford dictionary defines the social compact as an implicit agreement among the members of a society to cooperate for social benefits. From the perspective of natural selection favouring reproductive success, survival drops with the ability to reproduce in most species. But humans have an extended childhood and a long post reproductive stage. Davison and Gurven (2022) suggest that this potential for long life is an evolved feature of the life course, where the older generations, particularly grandparents, enable their own children to have more children. They suggest that humans as social animals have developed interdependence beyond kinship. For instance, humans value the promotion of skills in the younger generations because of some of the resulting productivity will be helpful to their generation and, in the longer run, for human life history.

Lifelong learning can be life-changing for individuals and enriching for societies. The social compact links generations through adaptations to the living context through learning. There is a saying that it takes years to have an overnight success. It is based on aggregating knowledge until the totality finally yields the answer that was sought in order to fit a societal need. It might be described in today's terms as societal 'crowd sourcing' of knowledge.

S. Brink, *The Longevity Dividend*, International Perspectives on Aging 39,
https://doi.org/10.1007/978-3-031-35335-2_9

9.2 The Social Compact for Societal Knowledge

The social compact governs the relations between people and social action for collective welfare and social benefit. It is an implicit agreement that governs shared assets, values and rules of behaviour across time. This compact covers many domains, of which knowledge is a key one. The social compact codifies the arrangements for the acquisition and exchange of knowledge between individuals as well as the collective ownership of knowledge (Manyika et al., 2020). It ensures that the use of such collective knowledge is directed to social progress and welfare of the population over time. Therefore, it is important to understand the role of individuals in relation to knowledge and their membership in a society and time: first, as a lifetime member of the individual's cohort in relation to other cohorts in a living generation, second, as a member of the individual's generation relative to past and future generations and finally as a member of the species.

Complying with the social compact ensures the collaboration of people of all ages over time in the production, use and consumption of knowledge for the greater good. This implies a shared desire for societal advancement, which motivates the members of society to cooperate based on expectations, responsibilities and processes for mutual and collective benefit through general will. If so, people privilege collective interest over purely personal interests for the betterment of the society in which they live (Rousseau, 2012).

9.2.1 Social Progress Through Knowledge Accumulation

The social contract that has evolved around knowledge as a public good is unique. The pool of human capital developed through knowledge accumulation leads to increases in economic growth and social development – a result of increased productivity and innovation, increased labour, greater social wellbeing, civic participation and social equity (Kenton, 2022). Such societal progress and welfare generation is dependent on continually increasing or improving human knowledge, which can be applied to evolving demands and new challenges. Lifelong learning of each generation is a key element for knowledge accumulation.

What motivates the accumulation of societal knowledge? According to the formulators of the theory of social contracts, three conditions need to be met (Neidleman, 2012). First, motivated by self-interest, individuals will follow the contract only if they benefit from social collaboration. This condition is easily met, because no individual, no matter how educated or wise can hold all the necessary knowledge to meet the challenges of society at all times. Would an individual be moved to shun lifelong learning by a desire to contribute less to the collaboration? This is unlikely because the knowledge one accumulates is the resource harnessed to get the most from one's life. An individual's stock of knowledge may depreciate or appreciate depending on their level of investment in learning. Besides, learning also has an intrinsic value independent of its transactional value in collaboration.

A second condition proposes that the welfare of others is a motivator only if the advantages an individual expects to derive depend on being willing to accord the same advantages to the individual's counterparts. Societal benefits arise from all the appropriate resources held by different individuals at the needed time coalescing into a critical mass to address a societal issue that could affect everyone. The cumulative integrated knowledge generates new concepts, ideas and practices that are essential for social institutions to improve lives through social innovation and action. The third condition is that the compact has to be seen as just and reasonable. The social compact for continuous knowledge acquisition and transmission is inclusive. It impels individuals to carry out their responsibilities, on the one hand, and protects them from being excluded or being left behind, on the other.

The Bonding of Generations Through Knowledge Continuity Under the Social Compact

Humans are exceptional in their ability to record, disseminate, exchange and evaluate the stock of knowledge and also to continually upgrade and add to it so that all members can benefit. The compact exemplifies the idea of knowledge reciprocity, which extends both between and within generations. Social networks and intergenerational interaction are essential for healthy living of individuals and social cohesion of societies. The sharing of knowledge through generations ensures that there is continuity both of learned experience and knowledge. Some indigenous societies have a 'knowledge keeper' responsible for preserving knowledge and transmitting it to the next generation. In oral societies, collective memory was built through recitations and songs, often originating with unspecified earlier generations. Written records codify known knowledge and the history of experiences that both benefited and disadvantaged societies.

9.2.2 *The Social Compact Manages the Stock and Flow of Knowledge*

Knowledge is a unique form of capital, unlike, say, financial capital. According to Stiglitz (1999), knowledge creates value in a critically different way from other forms of capital. This is because it can be expanded more easily and cheaply, and it can provide lucrative returns even when it is abundant. Sharing knowledge does not reduce its value to the sharer or to society. Individuals use their knowledge in work and in society as knowledge workers. Wise consumers make sustainable choices through their demand for products and services with increased knowledge embedded in them. Innovation and invention are people products, because human capital, even though it can be recorded and stored, is largely held and applied creatively by people.

Human capital, based on knowledge, is a form of intangible wealth. The stock and flow of knowledge connect to the demand and supply of knowledge. A simple explanation based on scientific literature can describe stock of human capital thus: The stock of human capital is the existing level of knowledge in a group (country, workforce) or an individual at a particular time. It is often expressed as the assessed value of a defined and accepted indicator of knowledge, such as a metric of literacy, education attainment or performance. When it refers to the average individually held knowledge rating in the country, it can be expressed as human capital per capita, which would be an estimate (since human capital held by similar persons can vary). The knowledge stock held can change over time as some of it becomes obsolete or forgotten, while new information may have been added.

The idea of change over time is captured in the concept of flow of human capital, which is the rate at which the knowledge level is being increased (or decreased) for a defined group over a given period of time. Change can be measured by comparing the stock at various time periods for a specific group of persons or by calculating the marginal change over successive time periods. The flow captures the amount of human capital being produced or added to human capital stock. The value of the human capital stock held by an individual is the basis for the concept of 'brain drain', when a highly educated individual leaves his home country for another as part of transnational human capital flow.

The flow and stock concepts are important for understanding the utilization of knowledge for the progress of society. In addition to preparing the individual members to function successfully in contemporary society, new knowledge additions to the stock prepare them to face new or unexpected challenges in their lifetime. This continuously adds cognitive capacity of both content and process, which enables future generations to do the same.

This systemic view of the knowledge process is managed at the individual level by widely accepted practices and processes, which also evolve over time. They complement many kinds of formal education, such as initial education or work-related training, whether compulsory or voluntary, and also lifelong learning, whether formal, informal or experiential. Because of the importance of this asset, societies invest in education and learning for individual members.

9.2.3 A Culture of Lifelong Learning Is Enabled by the Social Compact

The social compact embeds learning into living through a lifelong learning culture. What does a lifelong learning culture entail? Society's relationship to knowledge and learning is entrenched in culture, as is art or language. Knowledge and learning become enjoyable and valuable to both individuals and collective society.

A culture change is a societal mission that can only be achieved if everyone works jointly to achieve this goal. The United Kingdom formalized such change as a worthwhile coherent vision for a national popular culture, with shared responsibility for achieving it (Fryer, 1997). The societal mission to implement a lifelong learning culture requires a partnership between individuals and society and between private and public entities. The rapid pace of knowledge growth, and its embeddedness in every sphere of life, underlines the need for learning in every societal role such as worker, entrepreneur, parent and citizen. Everyone needs to be involved with learning, as learners, teachers, supporters and mentors, enabling individuals, families and communities to keep pace and develop together. An individual benefits from not only the human capital that is amassed during life, but also from living among people with valuable human capital and who are also learners that continuously gain more knowledge assets.

Lifelong learning by individuals is envisaged as a routine part of everyday activities practiced throughout life for growth, wellbeing and development. The currency and value of knowledge are global, so it can be acquired locally and internationally. A culture of lifelong learning starts with a transformed view of the knowledge held by individuals, which affects their daily life. It also expresses the collective power of society to improve the progress of each member for the advancement of all. Individuals are free to determine their own needs, select their own priorities and options and choose the means for and timing of their learning. This requires individuals to look for the quality, currency, validity and reliability of what they learn. Learning will open both minds and doors, without confining learning activities to particular times, places, forms or methods.

Citizens understand that, unless they exercise their responsibilities related to learning, they cannot count on the benefits of opportunities and success in society. In return, citizens can expect a coherent lifelong system of learning opportunities, which they can navigate to form their own pathways to personal learning goals according to their needs in life. Society and its institutions should reward competence and experience gained through learning.

The Social Compact Positions Each Society and Its Members for International Action and Global Citizenship

In an increasingly globalized world, learning has taken a planet-wide perspective. Knowledge can be developed in and spread from any part of the world through the internet and other media. Digital international service connections facilitate interrelationships with unknown others. The state of the world becomes a local concern, and people gain a world perspective on issues such as the health of the oceans and climate change. Learning promotes global citizenship of individuals not as spectators but as active contributors. Participation in international organizations through membership and financial support creates actors in transnational civil society, which generates further on-going learning.

9.3 Rights and Responsibilities for Learning of Individuals Under the Social Compact

The rights to and the responsibilities for learning extend through life. They ensure that the social compact supports the collective acquisition, ownership and transmission of knowledge and that the compact delivers the societal benefits that arise from this knowledge. All members of society can over time avail themselves to the right to lifelong learning and are, in turn, expected to carry out their responsibilities to themselves and contribute to improving the human condition.

9.3.1 The Right to Learning and Its Benefits Throughout Life

The citizenship right to learning governs the relationship between the individual and collective knowledge, including the production, management and use of human capital for both the personal and the common good.

The right to learning, particularly through public education, has been codified since December 10, 1948 through the UN Universal Declaration of Human Rights, Article 26 (United Nations, 1948). Lifelong learning is implied through the statement: 'Everyone has the right to education'. Education is considered a key social right along with the rights to housing, food and social security because knowledge is important for everyone to make the most of their lives. In addition, learning enables access to other social rights. Learning makes individuals well rounded and productive, which benefits not just themselves. It benefits also the economic, social and cultural development of the societies in which they live through the sharing of knowledge assets and their use. Thus, the second clause of Article 26 suggests that such learning should be directed to the full development of the human personality and to promote understanding of and collaboration between countries. The goal is democratic education provided to all societal members and to improve their competency to understand the world.

Democratic education is equally distributed learning opportunities for knowledge that meets the needs of individuals and society. The signatory states have an obligation to respect and fulfill this right for their citizens. By delivering learning as a democratic right, they gain an engaged and informed citizenry that can find their own productive paths to a better life through knowledge and to perform proficiently for the greater good of society.

The UNESCO Convention against Discrimination in Education from 1960 may hold states accountable for violations of the right to education both through acts of commission or omission. Objective criteria of availability, accessibility, acceptability and adaptability (so called 4 As) would be used for judging compliance (United Nations, 1999).

9.3.2 Individual Responsibility

Each individual is responsible for managing, maintaining, using and sharing knowledge for their entire life course. This responsibility relates both to knowledge gained from previous generations and knowledge gained through personal lifelong learning. They both contribute to human capital. The human capital amassed is a major asset for the individual, and it affects life opportunities, social mobility and professional success. Even if individuals are not motivated to invest in something bigger than themselves by bequeathing their knowledge for the greater good, enlightened individual self-interest is likely to prevail.

Individuals are responsible for using the stock of societal knowledge wisely, enhancing it for the current context and ensuring that this heritage will be in turn passed to future generations. To manage this responsibility, the individual must evaluate both concrete and abstract, tacit and explicit knowledge gained from previous generations. Such confirmed knowledge enriches individual lives in contemporary times. This is based on time tested values, which guide decision making and priority setting during good and hard circumstances. The successful response to new and unforeseen situations could be a blend of inherited information and new information from the current context. Change can be managed by relying on reasoning and problem solving of identified related issues, on procedures that identify internal and external impact factors and on codified experiential evidence about the processes and techniques that work.

To exercise their responsibility, individuals must demonstrate agency to hone their own skills of learning-to-learn and to learn throughout life. Such actions can maximize their potential and improve their own life achievements and the quality of life of their household. This would require willingness to accept the importance of expectations and standards set by society and to strive to make full use of societal arrangements (Haskins, 2009). Only individuals can determine their specific needs at different points in their life course for successful functioning in society. Doing so enables them to manage learning for their personal development.

By managing their learning, individuals can define the purpose of their learning, develop productive habits of learning and determine how they will wield the knowledge gained to meet the challenges of life. Managing their learning helps individual decision making about the choice of learning opportunity, the level of effort, and the time and financial investment required to gain the most in relation to their own capacity. It facilitates the maximal use of evidence for wise decisions and the choice of valuable traditions that would add meaning to life. This can include not only the enhancement of personal contributions during individuals' own prolonged lifetime, but also the transmission of their knowledge and experience to immediate family and descendants to enhance the future of the younger generations.

9.3.3 Generational Responsibilities

Societal knowledge is a crucial form of generational wealth. The cumulative human knowledge links generations over time for human development and societal progress. Continual improvements follow from both the interdependency between successive generations and the perpetuation of the continuously validated culture of learning. Therefore, each individual also has a generational responsibility to ensure intergenerational transfers.

Knowledge enriches generations in two ways. It does so, first, by enabling the knowledge assets of all cohorts to be increased and used for the benefit of the living generation. Exposure to the same learning stimulus does not, however, ensure equal results among individuals because of multiple individual and social intersectionality factors. Learning results in varying outcomes depending on when, where and how learning occurred, the open mindedness to new sources and methods of learning and the foundation to which new learning was added. Still, the diversity of individual knowledge and experience is an advantage when it is assembled as a common good. The sharing of individual knowledge communally builds capacity for joint action and social cohesion.

Second, knowledge enriches generations by means of evaluating, improving and amassing valid knowledge for the progress of future generations. Each generation is responsible for the acquisition, creation, organization, distribution and storage of knowledge to ensure that the knowledge stock is available for future users. Discontinuity or loss can be extremely detrimental to progress. For example, the loss by fire of the ancient Alexandria library is sometimes blamed for a knowledge setback of several centuries. Because knowledge benefits people everywhere, local knowledge exchanges expand to a global network of knowledge, albeit conditioned by the speed of dissemination, content relevance and assimilation of the distributed knowledge. Lessons of history and of societal mistakes can be exchanged. Some knowledge can be used infinitely and anywhere, forming the foundation for further development through science and invention.

9.4 The Learning Infrastructure Should Facilitate the Exercising of Individual and Generational Responsibilities

The lifelong learning system is under continuous construction. The system lags behind in meeting societal demands for an educated population. The task is complex and difficult because the history of the learning infrastructure has not been a straight line. Early learning infrastructure was developed for a minority of elites. The idea of universally available education is relatively recent. Efforts were made to make education widely accessible but with uneven results. Education for children was made compulsory in most countries. Understanding the transformative value of education for poverty eradication and social and economic development, many countries signed on to the global UNESCO-led movement 'Education for All' in 2015. However, the focus on the quantity of education resulted in mass education or the industrialization of education, and the quality of educational results suffered. Much of the infrastructure was directed to specific early stages of life, such as preschoolers and youth. Meanwhile, the speed of new knowledge creation continues to grow, which requires that citizens be able to gain necessary knowledge and skills to function well in modern society. This requires more of a lifelong learning perspective.

The lifelong learning infrastructure has to meet the learning requirements of all ages simultaneously in a continuously evolving economic, social and cultural context. The requirements for an efficient lifelong learning system are rapidly evolving, too. For successful learning, different pedagogies, various resources and exercises and multiple modes may be required. The desirable learning outcomes are not only evolving fast but also entail great diversity of knowledge and deep skills of critical thinking and problem solving. Individuals have to acquire the knowledge to balance and perform different life roles well, such as worker, parent and citizen, and which have to be performed concurrently. Learning outcomes now consist of content or expertise, on the one hand, and also learning-to-learn to enable regular additions to learning and skills, on the other.

Because every individual will be engaged in learning, the learning system is generally a whole-of-society effort. The scale and complexity of the learning sector requires provision of learning to be multi-sectoral, spanning the public, private and non-profit domains. Provision for learning requires multiple actors, such as agencies, institutions, private companies, teachers, instructors and tutors, that function individually and together to meet needs and demand. Advances in digital connectivity allows provision of learning to be international as well, ensuring that a learner can choose the best available learning option.

As the population ages, society is expected to provide opportunities for late-life learning for increasingly older learners. Governments have a key role to play. Their policies can support components of infrastructure, fund institutions, subsidize learners, and ensure quality and accreditation. Governments also monitor and evaluate the successes of the learning system. (See also Table 8.1).

9.4.1 Ensuring Equity and Quality in Learning Throughout Life

Global standards of competencies are in demand. They can require learners to be not only consumers of knowledge through life but also critical thinkers, innovators and knowledge creators using their knowledge. In managing efficient change in the lifelong learning system, societies face a dilemma. On the one hand, the current system has to be modernized and its quality improved and, on the other, it has to be extended to include learners in later life. Generic learning options, which serve the majority of learners, must be complemented with options that serve the particular needs of groups of learners. Examining the options for change through the prism of the needs of later learners can be a way to test the fairness of the current system and the alternatives.

9.4.2 Designing Lifelong Learning Options That Include Learners in Later Life

People in later life are not exempt from the rights and responsibilities of the social compact. It would be unfair to set high expectations for the reciprocity and outcomes of contributions of this cohort if the opportunities to meet their learning needs are absent or inadequate. The learning options can be examined relative to their individual and generational responsibilities.

Intention may differ from reality in the area of learning in later life. The extension of longevity has progressed faster than the development of infrastructure for learning for this late phase of life. While generic learning possibilities for all adults may be available, their particular needs are not always met. This population segment has learners with individual and multiple specific needs, which makes the diversity of needs so extensive that age can be an irrelevant descriptor of need. Lifelong learning by individuals in later life under current arrangements can be lacking, inadequate or, at least, uneven. In these circumstances, the later life cohorts may find it difficult or impossible to carry out their responsibilities under the social compact.

To reprise, the first responsibility, directed to benefit the individuals themselves and their families, includes the wise use of consolidated societal knowledge. In addition, they are expected to incorporate validated new knowledge and experience to add to cumulative human capital and to transmit this legacy to the next family generation.

Today's cohorts in later life have experienced a century of turbulence and prosperity. There have been world wars, economic recessions and booms, vital increases in health and quality of life, a couple of global pandemics and the growth of digital technologies. Late in life they are experiencing the existential threat of climate change and transitions to a new system of global alliances and evolving social structures. Some changes have been smooth, while others have been abrupt or disruptive. All changes have nonetheless influenced progress by slowing, redirecting or advancing it. Learning makes it possible for individuals to understand such past life events and to use opportunities to develop the path forward for their families and their future selves.

With a lifetime that can extend eight decades or more, today's older people have experienced exceptional change. The same can probably be expected for tomorrow's older people. Engaging in lifelong learning and continuous skills improvement are important for successful aging in these circumstances. This requires inherited knowledge to be continually tested against the contemporary context to distil the key values, knowledge and skills. Some people in later life view the lessons of life as learning opportunities and search out options that widen their contextual knowledge. Each generation is a memory bank that holds a store of learned knowledge vetted by experience and captured in family stories, language lore, rituals and traditions. The later learners are well positioned to benefit from improved quality of life and to pass on a legacy to the next generation.

The link to the previous generation could trace the family history and, if available, genetic heritage involving health and disease. It could describe change experienced over time through upward (or downward) mobility by parents, grandparents and even great grandparents. The evidence can be partial or complex, involving multigenerational networks or extend only to the previous generation. The history of growth and loss provides vital information on how skills and knowledge were orchestrated to meet the challenges and opportunities that were encountered. Family history can inspire by recognizing latent talent or redirect by identifying actionable ideas. It can also create the need for a completely new trajectory for future progress, based on the patterns of success and failure. Much anecdotal evidence from older learners shows they revive or develop an interest in their heritage to know who they really are, to understand who they have become and what they can contribute to the next generation. Butler (1963) suggested that people in later life universally start to examine their life as a whole in relation to the past as they recognize their own part in carrying forward the family history.

Their second generational responsibility is for individuals to invest in something larger than themselves and even to contribute to the betterment of future generations. Learners in later life add to the collective human capital of their own generation, identify knowledge that is no longer relevant and also detect over-the-horizon issues that are emerging. Sharing experiences of plausible scenarios can ease the transitions that members of the next generation are beginning to face.

To fulfill the generational responsibilities, lifelong learning must extend to include late-life learners. The process of educating the whole person starts in childhood and should continue through life. A learner-centric, demand-led customized approach to learning would be essential to respond to the range of needs of the diverse population segment of late-life learners. Features attractive to older learners include reality-based situations and use of their own knowledge and experience. Stimulating research of verifiable evidence and building capacities are also attractive features. Such capacities include the facility to understand and evaluate new information, the ability to use new technology and the skill to explain and use new learning. To attract people in their later years, learning options must be responsive to these learners' needs both in content and in how they are provided.

Learners in late-life are a growing population segment, so learning must keep pace with both their growth in numbers and the increase in knowledge. Providing up-to-date knowledge about the demands of everyday life in the world they live in is necessary if they are to discharge their roles and responsibilities. Becker (2002) estimated that 70% of the total national output in the United States is found in the human capital of people. This large percentage indicates the importance of human capital for national growth and progress. Learning inequities among and between age cohorts regarding both access to and provision of knowledge have been tolerated in the past. Large numbers of the older population operate without essential information for daily life. The impact of information asymmetry in society on the progress of the economy and society is accepted but unmeasured.

The later life stage should be part of a coherent lifelong system of learning opportunities. Late-life learners should be able to navigate the system to form their own pathways to personal learning goals throughout life, consonant with both their own needs and those of society. There are no established syllabi or course catalogues setting out the material to be learned for the older age cohorts, nor are structures set up for their learning. The immense diversity within the population after seven decades or more of life is part of the reason for this. Older people should be able to decide not only what they want to learn and when, but also how to gain access to the chosen learning option among the opportunities and modalities available. They will decide on the personal balance between formal, non-formal and informal learning. The consequences of their choices are important for their ability to manage the challenges of their lives through the knowledge gained. For this reason, they need to judge whether they can validate the quality and level of the transmitted knowledge. Some late-life learners may see value in their learning being formally accredited regardless of the learning institution and time of learning.

Both advantages and disadvantages are associated with the choice of learning opportunities. They relate to individual needs, the context, personal abilities, experience and the range of available options. For example, independent learning can be satisfying to an autonomous person with a wide network and the skills to seek out information. However, it may yield poor outcomes for someone who is isolated, has poor literacy and has several difficulties in managing learning. In other words, the benefits resulting from a specific learning option may vary because of the inherent characteristics of both the learning option and the late-life learner.

9.5 The Social Compact Links Longevity, Lifelong Learning and the Longevity Dividend

The social compact reflects values and shapes commitments for the shared aspirations of society. It transcends being a mere framework for transactions. It is culturally embedded so it generates social progress by collective action within and between generations. The social compact celebrates the achievement of greater longevity, and it includes the older generations as a vital part of society. Building a legacy of knowledge is a cumulative and collaborative societal process for achieving advancement between successive generations.

The member countries of the United Nations recognize the transformational potential that learning has for attaining sustainable collective futures captured in a new social contract that includes education (International Commission on the

Futures of Education, 2021). Without lifelong learning the continued upward trajectory of progress can be threatened. However, participation in learning activities tend to wane after initial education. This tendency needs to be remedied. Seeking to ensure that adults continue to learn, the European Union set a headline goal that 60% of all adults should participate in training by 2030 (European Commission, 2021). This would be an increase from 37% in 2016. Achieving compulsory education for all school age children is a goal in most countries. There are generally no promotions of learning or targets for participation in later life.

Longer lives add more years of shared knowledge and experience, which adds to the benefits that present and future society will reap from greater longevity. Amalgamating knowledge from a long-lived diverse population will broaden the base for tacit and explicit knowledge and experience harvesting. The anticipated impact will be larger than if drawing on a limited, homogeneous and short-lived population. The exercise of personal and generational responsibilities related to knowledge by this large population segment can lead to large economic and social gains for society. Longevity enriched by learning will be a blessing rather than a problem.

Achieving greater societal gains also requires society to take a life-course perspective for lifelong responsibilities and contributions, so as to ensure a just and fair transition to the desired future of the population as a whole. Collective human capital governs the design and achievement of the shared destiny of the population. A learning society of citizens can exercise their responsibilities and make societal contributions during their prolonged lives. The value of lifelong learning will therefore rise along with growth in the ability to manage the collective destiny through knowledge.

A widely accepted social compact will drive a cohesive societal effort through learning to achieve progress that benefits all equitably in living generations and future ones. Members of all cohorts should be active learners, not just spectators. If lifelong learning is partial, uneven, of poor quality or excludes some population groups, the potential gains are reduced, which deprives the whole population of current and future benefits.

Social choices have to be determined and implemented during the limited time of the population transition. Societies will rely on the cohesive force of the social compact to energize multiple partners to work together to enrich the longevity dividend for the benefit of all living and future members of society. The large later life population segment can make an enduring contribution to economic and social gains, or it can significantly detract from such benefits. Lifelong learning is the catalyst that can make the difference between the opposing outcomes. Expectations of achievement resulting from a well-functioning social compact provide guideposts for a holistic, multi-generational and multi-outcome examination of societal gains from the longevity dividend.

References

Becker, G. S. (2002). The age of human capital. In E. P. Lazear (Ed.), *Education in the twenty-first century* (pp. 3–8). Hoover Institution Press.

Burke, E. (1790). *Reflections on the revolution in France*. Printed for J. Dodsley.

Butler, R. N. (1963). The life review: An interpretation of reminiscence in the aged. *Psychiatry, 26*(1), 65–76. https://doi.org/10.1080/00332747.1963.11023339

Davison, R., & Gurven, M. (2022). The importance of elders: Extending Hamilton's force of selection to include intergenerational transfers. *PNAS, 119*(28), 1–12. https://www.pnas.org/doi/10.1073/pnas.2200073119

European Commission. (2021, May 7). *Porto Social Summit: All partners commit to 2030 social targets* [News]. https://ec.europa.eu/social/main.jsp?langId=en&catId=89&newsId=10004&furtherNews=yes

Fryer, R. H. (1997). *Learning for the 21st century: First report of the National Advisory Group for Continuing Education and Lifelong Learning*. http://hdl.voced.edu.au/10707/30387

Haskins, R. (2009, July 31). *The sequence of personal responsibility* (Article). http://www.brookings.edu/research/articles/2009/07/09-responsibility-haskins

International Commission on the Futures of Education. (2021). *Reimagining our futures together—A new social contract for education*. UNESCO. https://unesdoc.unesco.org/ark:/48223/pf0000379707.locale=en

Kenton, W. (2022, July 12). *Human capital definition: Types, examples, and relationship to the economy*. Investopedia. https://www.investopedia.com/terms/h/humancapital.asp

Manyika, J., Madgavkar, A., Tacke, T., Smit, S., Woetzel, J., & Abdulaal, A. (2020). *The social contract in the 21st century* (Report). McKinsey Global Institute. https://www.mckinsey.com/industries/public-and-social-sector/our-insights/the-social-contract-in-the-21st-century

Neidleman, J. (2012, October 9). *The social contract theory in a global context*. E-International Relation. https://www.e-ir.info/2012/10/09/the-social-contract-theory-in-a-global-context/

Rousseau, J.-J. (2012). *Du contrat social* [The social contract]. Flammarion. (Original 1762)

Stiglitz, J. E. (1999). Knowledge as global public good. In I. Kaul, I. Grunberg, & M. A. Stern (Eds.), *Global public goods: International cooperation in the 21st century* (pp. 308–325). Oxford University Press.

United Nations. (1948). *Universal declaration of human rights*. https://www.un.org/en/about-us/universal-declaration-of-human-rights

United Nations. (1999). *Economic, social and cultural rights. Preliminary report of the Special Rapporteur on the right to education, Ms. Katarina Tomasevski, submitted in accordance with Commission on Human Rights resolution 1998/33* (E/CN.4/1999/49). Economic and Social Council. https://digitallibrary.un.org/record/1487535?ln=en

Chapter 10
The Longevity Dividend and Societal Transformation

10.1 Longevity Dividend – Hype or Promise?

How real is the potential for a country to gain from the longevity dividend? Interest has burgeoned in accurately tracing and quantifying the size of the longevity dividend and its relation to learning. Early estimates mainly focused on savings in health budgets. Estimating a total gain is more complex, given the number of factors and variables of each national context. However, there are indications that longevity is likely positively related to the gains from the longevity dividend. Productivity, in terms of GDP per hour worked, was found to be positively correlated with high life expectancy in high income countries (Franklin, 2018). Life expectancy is a more powerful determinant of national productivity than either the young or old age dependency ratios. Countries with similar life expectancy can have very different GDP per hour. Furthermore, education and health were found to be important channels to raise productivity. Rising life expectancy was found to raise the returns to education. A small cluster of countries have both high life expectancy and high GDP per hour (Fig. 10.1). They have better productivity than other countries with similar life expectancy. This shows that it is possible for a country to realize a large gain from the longevity dividend.

10.2 The Legacy of the Longevity Dividend

Society can benefit from the longevity dividend only if it embraces later life as a new stage of human life due to greater longevity, even though it challenges existing ideas of age and aging (Scott, 2021). The changes start with updating the biblical threescore years and ten to fourscore years and ten and understanding the attendant profound implication for how normal life is enjoyed for nine decades or more. To

S. Brink, *The Longevity Dividend*, International Perspectives on Aging 39,
https://doi.org/10.1007/978-3-031-35335-2_10

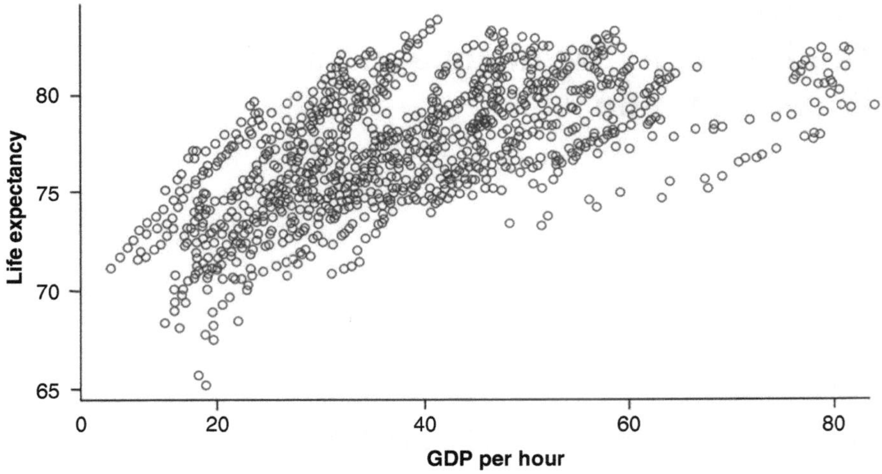

Fig. 10.1 Countries with the same life expectancy can have different productivity: life expectancy and GDP per hour (35 countries between 1970 and 2015). (Reproduced from Towards a longevity dividend: Life expectancy and productivity across developed countries by Franklin (2018) with permission from International Longevity Centre UK)

age in a society where a large share of the population is old is different from one where children's numbers dominated. The changes in social environment duly lead to prodigious change in individual behaviour, social structures and corporate and government policies. If they do not, the inaction will cast a long shadow over the future progress of the aging society. In contrast, instead of merely coping with the changes in the age structure of the population, the focus of the transition can become one that exploits the advantages of longer lives. Proactive societies can improve the aging process and integrate the roles of older people with society as a whole. For society to benefit from the longevity dividend in the long term, investments must have a life-course perspective.

The transition will change the way aging is viewed. The changes wrought by the longevity dividend will transform the way aging people live their lives and their importance in the public sphere. The malleability of aging means that long lives give individuals a longer horizon, a future ahead of them when they can delay, alter or re-order the sequence of commitments and life events. Changing social norms will reconfigure age-appropriate behaviour.

Societies will recalibrate the social contract and rework social institutions to stabilize the impact of the population transition. The cultural change accompanying the maturing of society will ensure that the normal process of aging occurs with no decline in rights but also in balance with the rights of younger generations and the reciprocal intergenerational relationships between them (Population Division, 2002). Such an adaption preserves the dignity and security of all stages of life, each with their rightful place in society. The success of this venture will determine if the longevity dividend will be an enduring gain for society and a benefit for all going forward.

10.3 *Projet de société* – A Whole of Society Long Term Effort for Societal Progress

The continuity of learning and the possibility of living longer than before are global characteristics of the twenty-first century. Jarvis (2008) suggested that if societies were serious about the value of learning because of its multiple benefits to society, a learning society must evolve to be a key factor in the incomplete project of humanity.

There is wide citizen support for making lifelong learning and education a priority. This holds regardless of individual characteristics or place of residence. In a survey covering seven million people from 194 countries, education was the top priority (United Nations, 2014). There is wide understanding that learning prepares people for solid employment and quality of life (UNESCO, 2021). There is an expectation that governments and the private sector should work together to provide opportunities for lifelong learning and skills development for adults.

Though lifelong learning as a concept has been discussed for years, its implementation has the characteristics of social innovation. Social innovation is the application of new ideas to create a novel solution to intractable social problems. The success of social innovation is indicated by its effectiveness, efficiency, sustainability and fairness compared to previous or existing solutions (Phills et al., 2008). The outcomes from social innovation are economic and social returns with benefits accruing to society as a whole rather than only to private individuals. They rely on multiple actors, both professionals and groups, in public and private sectors who use a variety of social processes and systems (Oeij et al., 2019). Torfing (2012) considers that interaction between private and public actors in innovation makes the problem definition sharper, generates better ideas and also instils a sense of ownership in solutions that are both new and bold.

Social innovation can drive a *projet de société*, which can be understood as a large, multidimensional, publicly supported long term societal effort to advance from aspirational to achievable goals. It is undertaken when the traditional models require fundamental change. This effort could include a cultural change that incorporates the benefits of both increasing longevity and lifelong learning. A key way to accomplish this is to develop the ethos and the supporting structures that create a longer productive life course and advance societal progress through knowledge.

The potential for public commitment to lifelong learning is high. This is because the change to living longer is universal, and the desire to increase the flow of benefits to all of society into the future is incontrovertible. The combination of collective action and systemic responses melds longevity and lifelong learning into the social fabric, and they are no longer special extras or short-term exceptions.

Governments provide leadership and direction. A *projet de société* is accepted as a long-term continuous process, which is unaffected by changes in elected administrations. While governments can introduce policies and take a variety of actions, securing the intended results requires working with societal partners. The rate of progress and the achievement of greater longevity dividends will depend on all components working together for common goals. Each country will design its unique pathway and process consistent with its own context.

10.4 The Learning Curve of Life

A learning curve is a meaningful concept for both individuals and society. It represents a process of continuous improvement over time due to learning ways to more effectively access knowledge. For individuals, it means learning-to-learn for each life stage, including in later life. This enables them to benefit from the process of lifelong learning. For societies, it means that, during the population transition, there is time and space to transform the lifelong learning ecosystem for better learning outcomes. The transformed system will continue to serve the future generations through life subsequent to the shift. The learning curve allows some latitude to examine the best options for the components and their linkages in the lifelong learning infrastructure. It also facilitates scheduling the process of change such that no learner in any generation will be disadvantaged by the changes.

10.5 Potential Ideas for Peer Learning and Exchange Among Countries

Successful aging and lifelong learning pose unique challenges for the statecraft of governments because they require lifespan policies, multi-ministerial action and multiple partnerships. Policies need to be reformed based on evidence. A system of modernized policies that are coordinated, synergistic and interoperable must be introduced for nation building for several future generations. Some countries have gained valuable experience from initial policy reforms and programs that could benefit other countries through peer learning. A few selected early examples of reforms, comprehensive policies and partnerships for successful aging and lifelong learning are described.

10.5.1 Production, Integration and Dissemination of National Data on the Aging Population

All countries have some kind of census and some also have other regular surveys. The data about the aging population can vary in thoroughness. Research to create evidence on the older population is often based on small or convenience samples and cannot provide reliable national data. Many countries cannot report in detail about the population aged sixty-five to a hundred years. Stakeholders would understand the rationale for national policies better if they were presented with a full statistical picture of the entire population. In most countries, much of the census information disseminated to the public still uses the category 'sixty-five and over' even though this group consists of as much as a fifth of the population. The Canadian statistical agency has started to report on the number and some characteristics of five-year age groups (cohorts) of people aged 65 to 100 years (Statistics Canada, 2023).

10.5.2 Research and the Creation of Evidence on the Changing Population Structure, Successful Aging and the Longevity Dividend

Research must record and analyze issues using data from the past but it must also address future topics. Press reports that signal newsworthy changes are useful but it is necessary to have rigorous research to sort out priorities. More research must focus on the momentous changes occurring among older people in an aging society in order to forecast future population needs. Solid evidence increases the chances of successfully enriching the longevity dividend and post priori evaluation can measure its impact. For example, researchers at numerous universities and organizations around the world are involved in useful research on topics related to the dividend. Some examples are reviewed by Lee and Mason (2011) and Franklin (2018).

10.5.3 Strengthening Enabling Legislation to Cover the Life Course

A substantive evaluation of the impact of a country's enabling legislation is essential to ensure that it applies over the full life course of all individuals without contradictions and that all policies can meet their national objectives. This is particularly the case since, despite the UN Universal Declaration of Human Rights, discrimination on grounds of age is not specifically prohibited. While older people require protection against violation of their rights, they also require guaranteed access to their benefits, such as the right to medical care, lifelong learning and equal outcomes of procedural and social justice. Some countries have acted to remedy this omission. For example, in the Constitution of Kenya, 2010, Article 27(4) prohibits discrimination directly or indirectly on sixteen grounds, specifically including age (Kenya Law, 2023).

10.5.4 Review of Existing Policies to Inform Modernization Strategies

Current social and economic policies were mostly developed during an earlier stage of population growth and are not ideal to meet the needs of the coming decades. An evaluation of existing policies in relation to current needs would expose policies that are no longer adequate and also gaps in the existing policy mix. A pension policy that provides incentives for early retirement is an example of a policy that is no longer suitable. Early retirement policies could be replaced by policies that provide flexible retirement options and incentives for working beyond age 65. New Zealand has had enviable success in its policies for older workers. Older workers form about a third of the New Zealand workforce and half of older workers aged 65 to 69 are employed. After review in 2022, New Zealand released 'The older workers employment action plan', with eleven action items to support older workers (Office of Seniors, 2022). A report by PwC UK (2018) found that the OECD countries as a whole would gain a potential long run increase of about US$ 3.5 trillion in the economy if they could increase older worker employment rates to New Zealand levels. The report suggests that supporting strategies for lifelong learning and retraining will be critical to achieving these gains. Work arrangements could also be reorganized to allow for part-time work, remote work and shorter work week options (Bussolo et al., 2015).

10.5.5 Comprehensive and Integrated Policies Address Needs in the Way They Are Experienced as Citizens Age

Current policy frameworks should be consistent with the population transition. A cohesive framework of policies allows older beneficiaries to combine them according to their needs and to adapt the combination of policies they use as their needs change. Multisectoral policies should address interrelated needs as they are experienced by individuals over their life course. The system should be easy to navigate and access seamlessly. They should be fair to all generations to support social solidarity. With greater longevity, an issue that affects a sizeable segment of older people is the risk of exhausting retirement savings just when the need for care and support rises in later life. Japan has introduced a comprehensive and integrated long term care insurance system, which supports aging at home, income security, preventive care, nursing, home care and long term care (Health and Welfare Bureau for the Elderly, 2016).

10.5.6 Incentives for Lifelong Learning

Though one cannot control the length of one's life, learning offers a strategy to prolong a life worth living. Learning is voluntary, and what and when an individual learns is therefore under the individual's own control. Those that engage in lifelong learning early tend to continue learning. While public education campaigns can promote lifelong learning, individuals need to experience economic and social benefits themselves in order to engage. For example, under Canada's Lifelong Learning Plan, an individual can temporarily use a certain amount of funds from a tax-deferral savings account when enrolled in full-time education (Government of Canada, 2023). The government of Singapore offers all individuals aged 25 and over an opening credit of S$ 500 to attend approved skills-based courses. This credit does not expire and there have been occasional top-ups (Government of Singapore, 2021).

10.5.7 A System That Encourages Learning Throughout Life

Some initiatives are making a start on the ideas in the aptly titled 'Sixty-Year Curriculum' (Dede and Richards, 2020). For example, Singapore initiated SkillsFuture in 2014 to give opportunities for development throughout life and incentives for lifelong learning while meeting the demands of Singapore of the future (Government of Singapore, 2023). Universities in Singapore support the upgrading of skills of their graduates over the long term. Graduates of some universities can take certain industry-relevant courses for 20 years after graduating or can have subsidized access to courses related to emerging skills. From 2021, universities and institutes offer free continuing education and training to their graduates in order to broaden skills (Government of Singapore, 2021).

10.5.8 Ensuring Opportunities in a Lifelong Learning Infrastructure

Though learning for pleasure and interest is valuable in itself, a greater return can be gained from learning that improves a person's quality of life, particularly in later life. A key challenge is to offer opportunities in a learning infrastructure accessible for all ages in all parts of the country. Early steps appeared to be age-based such as

Universities of the third age, rather than age-neutral learning opportunities. But some interesting approaches offer blended opportunities, sometimes with the objective of offering school learning to those who did not have that chance earlier in life. The Labour and Welfare Bureau and the Elderly Commission of Hong Kong introduced primary and secondary school education in Elder Academies in 2007, using existing institutions. Later they expanded these academies to include tertiary education when they found that many hoped to pursue university education or more specialized academic learning programs. There are about 190 Elder Academies in primary, secondary and post-secondary institutions in Hong Kong (Elder Academy, 2021).

In Korea, the different levels of government collaborate to support lifelong learning for citizens. For example, a network of more than 600 lifelong learning facilities in Suwon City (population 1.2 million) enables citizens to access a lifelong learning centre within a ten-minute walk (OECD, 2020). Suwon City won the UNESCO Learning City award in 2017. The country's fourth National Lifelong Learning Promotion Plan (2018–2022) encouraged learner centered learning in later life. Counselors and instructors were trained to help older people to plan their learning to achieve life satisfaction in their 'second life' or retirement (National Institute for Lifelong Education, 2018).

China has an extensive network of Open Universities with 45 branches and 3735 learning centers. To achieve national coverage for older learners, the Ministry of Education announced on November 2022 that the University of the Aged will operate with Open Universities (Du, 2022). People over 60 can learn foreign languages, computer skills, music, dance, photography, painting and other crafts and skills at these universities.

10.5.9 Better Outreach for Lifelong Learning by Collaboration with Partners

The strength of lifelong learning is that public efforts can be complemented by many potential partners: stakeholders, organizations, institutions and associations, professionals, tutors and digital instructors. Each such partner works with different groups and ages of learners and in a wide variety of venues and contexts. The involvement of civil society partners is vital for reaching vulnerable or disadvantaged learners. For instance, in Melbourne, Australia, Community Learning Champions work in culturally and ethnically diverse neighbourhoods in the inner city (Adult Learning Australia, 2023). They encourage neighbours and peers to use available learning and employment opportunities to improve their lives.

10.6 Later Life, Lifelong Learning and Productive Societies

Later life, lifelong learning and productive societies– these three factors are intricately intertwined. Managing them positively and constructively will result in benefits for citizens and the country. But the time available to accomplish this is limited and the time to act is now. The future hangs in the balance.

With better standards of living and improved health, life expectancy could extend healthy and active years of life to a hundred years or more. Life expectancy is expected to grow in this century in all countries but at different times and rates. Changes in life events and patterns of behaviour in prolonged lifetimes have had unanticipated economic, social and cultural impacts. Citizens are healthy, active and contributing members of society even in later life. How much a country benefits from greater longevity will depend on whether it is seen as an opportunity or as a problem.

Societies that consider greater longevity as a wonderful human achievement and work to benefit from the longer lives of citizens can gain the longevity dividend. The result is a productive society with greater economic benefits and social progress achieved during the population transition. The opportunity lasts only as long as the transition period from a society with a high proportion of children to one with a high proportion of older people. The longevity dividend derives from the shift to a population structure with a greater number of adults with knowledge and skills that contribute to society during longer lives. Societies can take advantage of this time limited transition by making strategic choices to enrich the longevity dividend. One strategy to increase the dividend is to increase the total contributions which benefit society that individuals make over their longer lifetime. The second strategy is to improve the value of these contributions. These strategies result in a productive society, where every citizen contributes throughout life for his or her own benefit and for society. When the entire population contributes to society during a longer lifetime, the country experiences accelerated economic growth and social progress that benefit current and future generations.

This outcome can be accomplished by ensuring lifelong learning for all citizens. The ideal lifelong learning system serves the entire population by continually incorporating new knowledge and responding to social needs over time. The resulting learning society thrives on creation, distribution and use of knowledge for the benefit of everyone. Lifelong learning of citizens improves their health and life outcomes through knowledge. Collectively, learners make more and better societal contributions for longer during their lifetimes.

Forward-thinking societies will re-imagine aging, incorporate learning into everyday life, create innovative technologies and redesign policies to accommodate greater longevity in society. If life lasts one hundred years, there are seventy-five or more years of life after most people complete their initial education. During that length of time the world will change dramatically and knowledge can grow astronomically. The world is going through green economy, geopolitical, climate and digital transitions at the same time as the population transition. Lifelong learning accessed by the whole population during the entire life course enables society to meet current and future challenges.

The window of opportunity and the urgency to act coincide in this case, which is a rare confluence. Moreover, and importantly, the solution is known. Forewarned is to be forearmed. Countries that understand the urgency will not squander this one-time opportunity. Because of the longevity dividend, the rewards that result from a commitment to lifelong learning compound over time. The consequences for the rest of the twenty-first century will therefore depend on timely societal choices. Countries that aged earlier or faster have demonstrated what is possible and mistakes to avoid. Those that prioritize lifelong learning provided valuable international experience and gained resulting initial benefits. When there is always an option for lifelong learning, a long life is enriched.

To long life!

References

Adult Learning Australia. (2023). *Lifelong learning for a fairer Australia: Champions for lifelong learning*. https://ala.asn.au/champions-lifelong-learning/

Bussolo, M., Koettl, J., & Sinnott, E. (2015). *Golden aging: Prospects for healthy, active and prosperous aging in Europe and Central Asia*. World Bank Group.

Dede, C. J., & Richards, J. (Eds.). (2020). *The 60-year curriculum: New models for lifelong learning in the digital economy*. Routledge.

Du, Q. (2022, November 17). China sets up national university for aged, to 'build lifelong learning society'. *Global Times*. https://www.globaltimes.cn/page/202211/1279845.shtml

Elder Academy. (2021, December 31). *About elder academy*. https://www.elderacademy.org.hk/en/aboutea/index.html

Franklin, B. (2018). *Towards a longevity dividend: Life expectancy and productivity across developed countries*. International Longevity Centre UK. https://ilcuk.org.uk/wp-content/uploads/2018/10/ILC-UK_-_Towards_a_Longevity_dividend.pdf

Government of Canada. (2023, February 22). *Participating in the Lifelong Learning Plan (LLP)*. Canada Revenue Agency. https://www.canada.ca/en/revenue-agency/services/tax/individuals/topics/rrsps-related-plans/lifelong-learning-plan.html

Government of Singapore. (2021, March 26). *Free continuing education and training modules for class of 2021 and 2020* (Press release). Ministry of Education. https://www.moe.gov.sg/news/press-releases/20210326-free-continuing-education-and-training-modules-for-class-of-2021-and-2020

Government of Singapore. (2023, 15 February). *Skills future*. https://www.skillsfuture.gov.sg/

Health and Welfare Bureau for the Elderly. (2016). *Long-term care insurance system of Japan*. Ministry of Health, Labour and Welfare. https://www.mhlw.go.jp/english/policy/care-welfare/care-welfare-elderly/dl/ltcisj_e.pdf

Jarvis, P. (2008). *Democracy, lifelong learning and the learning society: Active citizenship in a late modern age*. Routledge.

Kenya Law. (2023). *Constitution of Kenya, 2010*. The National Council for Law Reporting. http://www.kenyalaw.org:8181/exist/kenyalex/actview.xql?actid=Const2010

Lee, R., & Mason, A. (Eds.). (2011). *Population aging and the generational economy: A global perspective*. Edward Elgar and International Development Research Centre.

National Institute for Lifelong Education. (2018). *Lifelong learning in Korea. Volume 1* (PM2018-41). Korea. https://uil.unesco.org/system/files/2018_lifelong_learning_in_korea_vol.1.pdf

OECD. (2020). *Strengthening the governance of skill systems: Lessons from six OECD countries*. OECD Skills Studies. https://doi.org/10.1787/3a4bb6ea-en

Oeij, P. R. A., van der Torre, W., Vaas, F., & Dhondt, S. (2019). Understanding social innovation as an innovation process: Applying the innovation journey model. *Journal of Business Research, 101*, 234–254. https://doi.org/10.1016/j.jbusres.2019.04.028

Office of Seniors. (2022). *Older workers employment action plan*. Government of New Zealand. https://officeforseniors.govt.nz/assets/Uploads/Older-Workers-Action-Plan-FINAL.pdf

Phills, J. A., Jr., Deiglmeier, K., & Miller, D. T. (2008). Rediscovering social innovation. *Stanford Social Innovation Review, 6*(4), 33–43. https://www.gsb.stanford.edu/faculty-research/publications/rediscovering-social-innovation

Population Division. (2002). *World population ageing: 1950–2050*. ST/ESA/SER.A/207. United Nations. https://digitallibrary.un.org/record/461899?ln=en

PwC UK. (2018, June). *PwC Golden Age index*. https://www.pwc.co.uk/economic-services/golden-age/golden-age-index-2018-final-sanitised.pdf

Scott, A. J. (2021). The longevity society. *Lancet Healthy Longevity, 2*(12), e820–e827. https://doi.org/10.1016/S2666-7568(21)00247-6

Statistics Canada. (2023). *Data tables, 2021 Census of Population*. https://www12.statcan.gc.ca/census-recensement/2021/dp-pd/dt-td/index-eng.cfm

Torfing, J. (2012). Samarbejdsdrevet innovation i den offentlige sektor: Drivkræfter, barrierer og behovet for innovationsledelse [collaborative innovation in the public sector: Drivers, barriers and the need for innovation management]. *Scandinavian Journal of Public Administration, 16*(1), 27–46. https://ojs.ub.gu.se/index.php/sjpa/article/view/1565/1370

UNESCO. (2021). *The World in 2030. Public survey report*. https://unesdoc.unesco.org/ark:/48223/pf0000375950.locale=en

United Nations. (2014). *We the peoples: Celebrating 7 million voices*. My World. The United Nations Global Survey for a Better World. https://www.un.org/youthenvoy/wp-content/uploads/2014/10/wethepeoples-7million.pdf

Index

S. Brink, *The Longevity Dividend*, International Perspectives on Aging 39,
https://doi.org/10.1007/978-3-031-35335-2

M

N

MIX
Papier aus verantwortungsvollen Quellen
Paper from responsible sources
FSC® C105338

FSC
www.fsc.org

If you have any concerns about our products,
you can contact us on
ProductSafety@springernature.com

In case Publisher is established outside the EU,
the EU authorized representative is:
Springer Nature Customer Service Center GmbH
Europaplatz 3, 69115 Heidelberg, Germany

Printed by Libri Plureos GmbH
in Hamburg, Germany